14 FEB 1995
LONG LOAN

LONG LOAN
- 5 FEB 2007

13 MAY 1998
LONG LOAN

- 4 FEB 2002
LONG LOAN

17. DEC. 1976

3

85

2.

ONE WEEK

This book is due for return not later than the last date
stamped above, unless recalled sooner.

NO CHANGE

Wendy Cooper

NO CHANGE

A Biological Revolution for Women

Hutchinson of London

Hutchinson & Co (Publishers) Ltd
3 Fitzroy Square, London W1

London Melbourne Sydney Auckland
Wellington Johannesburg Cape Town
and agencies throughout the world

First published 1975
© Wendy Cooper 1975

Set in Monotype Baskerville

Printed in Great Britain by The Anchor Press Ltd
and bound by Wm Brendon & Son Ltd
both of Tiptree, Essex

ISBN 0 09 124080 8

'Though her years were waning,
her climacteric teased her like
her teens.'

Lord Byron DON JUAN

Contents

Foreword

by Sir John Peel KCVO FRCP FRCS

I am pleased to write a brief foreword to Wendy Cooper's book on the menopause, because, having read it with ease and interest, I am sure it will help a great many women who read it to have a better understanding of the many problems relating to their physical and mental health which occur at this particular time of their lives. Being written by a laywoman, it is in a language and style more easily understood and appreciated by a lay reader. The author has taken a quite remarkable amount of time and trouble to inform herself about the subject. She has visited clinics and specialists in Europe and North America as well as in Britain; she has spent hours on the telephone talking to doctors and victims; and shown a monumental degree of patience in reading letters received and in answering them. She has obtained the personal views of many gynaecologists and physicians, and faithfully recorded them and delved with unusual dedication into the literature.

The changes that affect both the body and the mind at and after the menopause are immensely complicated. Not only are there hormonal changes, but also emotional, social and family changes, and no one really knows why in fact some women, albeit the minority, pass through their fifties and sixties with little physical or emotional disturbance.

I am convinced from experience that Hormone Replacement Therapy can be of immense help to a great many women, but I am equally certain that it should only be made available under very strict medical supervision. Not only do we not know all about the biochemical interactions that take place when Oestrogen Replacement Therapy is given but we certainly do not know all the long-term side-effects.

If Wendy Cooper's book is widely read, as I hope it will be, it should do much to educate women about themselves and to stimulate them to seek medical advice instead of putting up with unpleasant and at times disastrous symptoms in the belief that they are the inevitable consequences of being a woman who must grin and bear it all.

The author's enthusiasm and dedication emerge from every page of the book, and if this leads her to over-simplification and even exaggeration at times this is no bad thing; such is the path the pioneer must tread. I wish this book every success.

J.P.

Introduction —
The choice is yours

Just once or twice in the life of a working journalist, there comes a story so exciting, important and demanding that it refuses to be written out or written off. You may present it in a dozen different ways for a dozen different papers and magazines. In the process *you* may become exhausted, but the subject does not. Instead of public interest and response declining, they increase. The law of diminishing returns fails to operate. In the end you have to recognize that instead of *you* running the story, the story is running you.

It has been that way for me with the story of Hormone Replacement Therapy (HRT) to eliminate the menopause. This revolutionary medical concept sees the menopause as a hormone deficiency condition, and sets out to treat it by replacing the declining oestrogen. Increasing numbers of women all round the world are already using it, and in 1971 I began intensive research both here and in America. I published the first series of articles entitled 'A Change for the Better' in April 1973 in the *London Evening News*. Since then there has been a continuous demand for major features on the same subject, for radio and television programmes and for talks; not just talks to women either, but sometimes, and surprisingly, to doctors.

Even when I have turned to other subjects, these have tended to be related, arising out of different aspects of the same research, and so HRT (by now we are on familiar terms) still found its way legitimately into several more general features on ageing. But it also insinuated itself far less predictably into features on show business ladies, on Women's Lib and even into a serious study on the status of women.

For over two years now the subject has dominated for me group discussion, private conversation and public talks. Even when *I* have decided that the occasion is not suitable, and that the words 'Hormone Replacement' shall not pass my lips, someone else has thought otherwise and brought the subject up. Once raised, no other subject has a chance. HRT just takes over.

And it has taken over at home too. For one thing it has acquired a vast physical presence. The files of reports, surveys and official medical papers are now too bulky to stand on the shelves and so cover the top of my desk. But the file I am most conscious of, which seems to sit there in mute reproach, is the one containing the letters I have received from women – over five thousand of them.

These letters make two things uncomfortably clear. First, that, despite the complacent attitude of a good many doctors, who insist that the menopause is only a *temporary* inconvenience and nothing to make a fuss about, there are, in fact, many women who suffer from it both acutely and for a long time. Secondly, they make clear that many women have no idea that any effective medical treatment exists.

So I have accepted what I must do. I must write this book. But the writing will not be an act of exorcism. HRT may have haunted, pursued and possessed me, but it is no pale ghost to be laid by the power of the word.

On the contrary, Hormone Replacement Therapy is a firm reality, a practical working treatment already changing the lives of countless women. What the book must do, therefore, is communicate this reality, and provide shape, form and detail. It must present the facts. It must look both at the female menopause, and at the therapy which makes it obsolete. It must weigh the advantages and disadvantages, analyse the support and the opposition. And it must do it where possible, in human terms, using case-histories, interviews and letters. Finally it must examine the implications and the future of this biological revolution, both for women and for society.

Although by its very nature, the book must be written with women in view, it must also have men in mind. For the truth is that it is not just women who suffer from the female menopause. Husbands and families suffer as well.

It must already be obvious that this cannot be an uncommitted book. Eight months after beginning my research, visiting medical centres, talking to gynaecologists, endocrinologists, and to hundreds of women, some of whom had been on oestrogen replacement for twenty years, I decided the weight of evidence justified my going on HRT myself. If I were to write about it, above all if I were to advocate it, as began to seem likely, I must be prepared to use it myself.

I was, of course, the right age. At fifty-one, I had already experienced two years of very odd symptoms, which at the time I had not even recognized as menopausal. But now from my researches it was clear these problems had been the early results of growing oestrogen deficiency. In my case, hot flushes were mild, but I was afflicted with riveting, violent pains in bones, joints and head, particularly when just dropping off to sleep. These were so severe that they jerked me even out of deep pill-induced sleep. Growing insomnia, depression and a deflating lack of confidence and decision completed a pattern entirely alien to my previous buoyant and rather positive nature. There were times when I really thought I was suffering from some frightful obscure disease, and throughout, though my young doctor was sympathetic, the word menopause was never mentioned and only mild tranquillizers and sleeping pills were prescribed.

Ironically by the time I knew enough about HRT to be prepared to use it, the worst of this phase of early glandular disturbance and imbalance had passed. But tests revealed I was extremely low in oestrogen and, alert by then to the long-term effects, I went onto HRT more or less as an insurance against future trouble, and in the hope of slowing down ageing processes.

Since that rather tentative decision back in 1972, my position has become firmer. Not only have I thrived on the treatment personally, but more and more evidence has continued to come in, not just concerned with the short-term effect of Hormone Replacement, in eliminating the common menopausal symptoms we are familiar with, but concerned with the long-term protection I was looking for against the deep-seated and unseen changes, known to be associated with oestrogen deficiency. And evidence has increased to indicate the protective role of oestrogen against some of the serious diseases, to which women become more vulnerable after the menopause.

My confidence has been boosted still further, by finding that not only in America, but in Britain as well, top men, men like Sir John Peel, the Queen's former gynaecologist, have been quietly using this therapy for their patients for many years.

So while this book must present all the medical, social and economic arguments both for and against HRT, to enable readers to make up their own minds, my own position will be clear.

It is quite simple. I believe there is a special charge on doctors and on modern medicine to bring effective help to women in relation to the menopause and the years that follow. It is, after all, modern medicine which has created the present situation, in which women in the developed world now live, on average, to around seventy-five years. That can mean a third of a life-time deprived of oestrogen. It is the duty of modern medicine to ensure that the extra years it has won for them are lived comfortably and fully, not crippled and limited by the effects of oestrogen deficiency.

I believe that women have the right to age in a way that parallels the ageing process of a man, with no abrupt decline, no accelerated ageing, and no atrophy of the sex organs to make intercourse painful, sexual response impossible, and middle-aged marriage a misery.

But the task of the book is really to set out the choice. The fact that women have such a choice, at last, is enough to make someone burst into print as well as into praise.

What can't be cured must be endured, and in the past women did just that. Now for the first time in history, where the menopause is concerned, they do not have to. They can decide for themselves if their menopause is really necessary. Some will still feel it is. They will reject on principle a routine which involves them in a daily pill, three weeks out of every four. Others, with only mild menopause symptoms, will also prefer to let nature take its course.

But there will be many who are suffering severely, and others who are simply motivated toward staying as young as possible as long as possible, who will feel that Hormone Replacement is for them. Still others will just derive benefit from the fact that a choice exists, from the knowledge that if things become too bad effective help can be given. The existence of the choice in itself springs the trap, reduces tension.

Many American women will already be familiar with Hormone Replacement Therapy both in concept and in practice. Some 80% of American gynaecologists already prescribe it, and one in three American women use it. For them the book will largely reinforce existing knowledge, both about the menopause itself and about the treatment, and bring together all the latest research findings and information.

For the British woman I hope the book will go some way toward redressing the balance. It will ensure that she too knows Hormone Replacement Therapy exists, how it works and the different oestrogens available, making the important distinction between synthetic oestrogens and naturally occuring oestrogens. It will also set out the latest variations in methods of oestrogen administration, in the length of cycles and the ways in which oestrogen on occasions is combined with other sex hormones, such as progesterone and testosterone, to meet individual needs.

Finally for every woman on both sides of the Atlantic, I hope this book will make clear that no longer, unless she chooses, need she be fobbed off during the menopause with prescriptions for palliatives such as aspirin, Librium or Valium, or worse still dismissed with the words, 'It's just your age. There is nothing to be done. You must put up with it.'

There is a great deal to be done. You don't have to put up with it. The choice is *yours*.

1. Biological Lib

Freud said 'Biology is destiny'. No woman is going to argue with that. They are all too familiar with the truth of it in their own experience. From puberty onwards women are constantly, in one way or another, the victims and the prisoners of their own biology.

But it is equally true in terms of the evolution of the human race. The fact that men, as young adults proved to be bigger, taller and stronger than women, not unnaturally enabled them to assume the dominant role. By contrast, female biology, the lighter physique, but above all the crippling limitations imposed by reproductive functions, prevented women from successfully challenging the existing situation – until now.

In the past the long, dangerous and weakening years of repeated child-bearing and caring kept women first from the hunting pack, and later from the councils of power. And it has gone on much the same way ever since, despite the female conceit (or is it crafty male deceit?) that 'the hand that rocks the cradle rules the world'. Except for a few exceptional women, most female hands have been too tired or too empty of gold to shape their own lives, let alone shape history. No wonder they have fallen back, all too literally, on the precarious politics of the bedroom, exerting oblique influence on men and events as and when they could.

And then in this century, tentatively at first and always in the face of opposition, women began to be given the chance to control the biology which had for so long controlled them. The first glimmerings of Biological Lib came with the better hygiene, better medical care and development of anaesthetics, which gradually reduced the danger and the pain of childbirth. It was Queen Victoria, too often and unjustly remembered only as a symbol of prudery, who gave anaesthesia respectability and impetus, by having chloroform administered for a royal birth, and so helped to defeat the sanctimonious 'against nature' lobby.

It was this same 'against nature' argument which in this century was raised again, first to oppose contraception and later to obstruct Hormone Replacement.

The battle for modern contraception has been won, and the old hit-and-miss methods have given way to the highly efficient and widely used intra-uterine device and the contraceptive pill. These techniques do not rely on suspect barriers, but enable women to manipulate and control their own biology. The IUD prevents any fertilized egg implanting itself in the wall of the uterus, and the contraceptive pill ingeniously raises the female hormone levels to simulate those of pregnancy, so that ovulation is prevented just as it would be in a real pregnancy.

So women in their fertile years have achieved for the first time the ability to control their own biology, to plan their families and their lives, and compete at last on something like equal terms with men.

But evolution has set another brake on female enterprise and energy, coming into operation in mid-life in the form of the menopause. More correctly the whole process of degeneration, starting with the atrophy and shut-down of the ovaries and continuing through to old age, is known as the climacteric. The menopause strictly means only 'final menstruation', but because it is accepted among women and in common parlance to have the wider meaning, the term is used in that sense also throughout this book.

So, with Biological Lib within the grasp of the younger woman who wants it, the same knowledge of the complex chemistry and workings of the sex hormones, which led to the development of the contraceptive pill, has now been used to bring about a second biological revolution, just as radical and profound for the older woman.

Most revolutions are designed to bring about change, this one is designed to prevent it, to prevent 'the change of life'. Again the concept is beautifully and ingeniously simple, and again it relies on artificially manipulating the female hormone levels.

It was known of course that the menopause came about as the result of the decline in the number of stored ova or eggs. Every girl baby is born complete with her generous endowment of potential ova, numbering several hundred thousand. But of these only some four hundred actually mature and once they are used up, that is that. Fertility is over. The ovaries respond to new instructions and begin to close down, so that the production of the two vital female sex hormones, oestrogen and progesterone, declines. The result is an irregular menstrual pattern and finally an end to the monthly cycle.

Unfortunately it is also the beginning of glandular imbalance and the familiar menopause symptoms. It is the beginning too of more deep-seated changes in the body which take place in the post-menopause years, and which come about due to lack of circulating oestrogen.

After the menopause, the ovaries become small and shrivelled, the lining of the womb atrophic and the vaginal skin thin and more vulnerable to infection. The vagina itself narrows and the external skin also becomes thin and less sexually responsive. The mucous membrane of the bladder also takes part in this pelvic atrophy, and the resultant thinning of the sensitive bladder neck contributes to the urinary frequency and urgency which sometimes occurs in older women.

The degenerative changes in the skin also show elsewhere, and loss of subcutaneous fat gives rise to extensive wrinkling, with the skin becoming dry, scaly and inelastic. Absence of oestrogen also causes breasts to become flabby, while the nipples flatten out and become non-erectile. It also permits a rise in bone resorption leading to thin and brittle bones (osteoporosis) in later years.

Obviously the shut-down and atrophy of the ovaries cannot be prevented, and there was never any question of restoring fertility. It could not be done and anyway most women in mid-life would not want it. What could be restored, and very simply, was the normal pre-menopausal level of oestrogen. If the wretched symptoms so many women experienced were really due to oestrogen deficiency, then restoring it should eliminate them. It did. In practice the concept was found to work exactly as the gynaecologists who pioneered it had predicted. Hot flushes were eliminated, vaginal atrophy relieved, and increased resorption of bone prevented. In fact the body was restored to pre-menopausal hormone balance and pre-menopausal harmony.

But it was one thing to prove that it worked, and quite another to get a traditionally minded medical profession to accept the revolutionary idea of the menopause as a deficiency condition that needed treating. After all, over the centuries the 'change' had been considered as a natural and inevitable part of ageing, a normal state for a woman at a certain time of life. No one ever bothered to consider the cause; in fact, age itself was considered cause enough, until modern endocrinology and a new understanding of hormones suggested otherwise.

The man in the forefront of the biological revolution to make the menopause obsolete, expounding the concept, putting it into practice and fighting to gain for it both acceptance and respectability, was a British-born gynaecologist, Robert Wilson, working in New York. As Consultant in Obstetrics and Gynae-cology at four big New York hospitals, he began his first investigations half a century ago.

He believed rightly that the menopause had been largely neglected by medicine because some women never develop serious problems; those who do and even dare to complain, are too often treated by doctors as hypochondriacs. There was some justification for the traditional view of the menopause as an unavoidable part of ageing, when nothing effective could be done to help. But Dr Wilson felt that the new discoveries should be changing these *laissez-faire* medical attitudes. He set out quite deliberately to shock what he called the 'nice-Nellies' of either sex, many of them doctors, by describing the meno-pausal women as 'castrates', deprived of sexual function. And he went on to draw a horrifying picture of the post-meno-pausal woman, liable to drying tissues, weakening muscles, sagging skin, brittle bones and shrinking vagina.

If there was an element of over-statement in all this, at least as shock tactics it worked. And by administering oestro-gens, first by injection and later orally, he proved that many of the changes believed to be an integral part of middle-age in women, could be prevented and even reversed. In fact part of his credo, imparted with almost messianic zeal, was that Hormone Replacement Therapy ideally should be seen as preventive medicine, to forestall the onset of the menopause before it even happened.

During the fifties and sixties, Dr Wilson not only put his

concept widely into practice, but kept up a flow of medical papers and articles on the subject, and finally set up the Wilson Foundation, a non-profit-making organization, dedicated to funding and inspiring both research and propaganda concerned with HRT. It was a stirring and successful crusade, and it culminated in 1966 with him becoming author of a best-seller called *Feminine Forever*, published in Britain by W. H. Allen and in America by M. Evans.

Dr Wilson's book was based strongly not only on his convictions and attitudes as a doctor, but on his convictions and attitudes as a man, betraying a romantic regard that amounts almost to reverence for that mysterious core of womanhood which he calls 'femininity'. This quality, a subtle blend of the sexual and emotional rooted deep in our correct hormone balance, could be, he believes, cruelly extinguished by what he terms the 'castrating' effects of the menopause, leaving a neutered and devalued creature, deserving man's pity rather than his passion.

Writing as a woman for other women, and also writing almost ten years later in the age of Women's Liberation, my own approach is inevitably less romantic and more rational, with perhaps less emphasis on femininity and more on feminism, and the right of women to more say in decisions medical or social, which affect their own bodies and their own lives.

Also, nothing as dynamic as Hormone Replacement Therapy, subject to wide use and wide research, can ever stand still, and some of the thinking and some of the details of technique have changed since Robert Wilson first launched his campaign and wrote his major papers. But his basic concept is still triumphantly vindicated by results, and when I met him in New York in March of 1972, I met a man whose battle was well on the way to being won on the American continent.

However, though he was then approaching seventy-five, he made it clear he would go on campaigning until full acceptance for HRT was achieved throughout the world, and most especially in his country of birth, Great Britain. He estimated then that it might be another ten years before the majority of the British medical profession were converted to the concept.

Although the majority of gynaecologists in the USA (figures suggest between 65% and 80%) are convinced advocates of HRT, there are also some who have reservations about long-term use and will only prescribe for short periods. At family doctor level, particularly in country areas, there is still resistance based on either apathy or ignorance.

Despite this, the United States leads the world in use of Hormone Replacement at the menopause, with Canada, South Africa and West Germany not far behind. After them come Italy, France, Brazil, Mexico and Japan, while Great Britain, incredibly for such a medically advanced country, is still somewhere at the bottom of the league, below even the tiny Phillipines.

But things are changing fast. More and more top British gynaecologists and endocrinologists are coming out in open support of HRT, with the inevitable result that this has on other more junior consultants and on family doctors, looking for a lead in the midst of the controversy.

Taking part with me in the popular BBC radio programme *You and Yours*, Dr Gerald Swyer, a leading British endocrinologist, who is consultant at University College Hospital, London, stated,

There are many women who from the menopause onwards experience significant deficiency of oestrogen. There is no question whatever that for them Hormone Replacement Therapy is the specially indicated treatment. Apart from relieving immediate symptoms, we have good reason to believe that much of the osteoporosis (brittling of bones) experienced by older women can be relieved by oestrogen replacement, and there is also a prophylactic effect against cardio-vascular disease.

The words of great men carry great weight and are powerful weapons in any war. This book will be quoting from many such authorities. But in the battle of Biological Lib, women themselves also have a part to play. To enable them to play it, they need to understand what the controversy is about and why it exists. And to do this, the role of oestrogen itself must be understood. For this hormone is the key to a woman's health and happiness, and it is at work in the body even before birth.

2. The role of oestrogen — the making of a woman

It is no exaggeration to say that the powerful female sex hormone, oestrogen, is crucial in forming and maintaining a woman, and it begins its work as early as six months before birth, to influence the growing foetus in the female direction.

Although oestrogen is totally essential to complete this differentiation, gender and sex are actually determined at the very moment of conception along with all other characteristics.

This marvellous mechanism of heredity is so inter-related with the action of oestrogen, and the two stories are so fascinating, compelling and interwoven, that I shall make no apology for combining them here.

When you consider the billions of people alive today, the great procession that has gone before and the vast numbers that will come after, it is not easy to accept the fact that there is no one in the world quite like you, never has been and never will be again. You are unique. And if you think that is a line in smooth flattery, you are wrong. It is the simple truth; a hard statement of scientific fact, rooted in the laws of genetics and mathematics.

The process is a curious mixture of the random and the precise. Nothing in the biological sense could be more random than the coming together of the two people who are to be the parents. Yet this one man and this one woman are each unique, carrying their own special blueprints, precisely written and coded on pairs of genes, which are strung like beads on the twenty-three pairs of chromosomes contained in each cell in the body.

There is just one special type of cell, the mature sex cells (the ova in the female and sperm in the male) which are different. In those there are only twenty-three *single* chromosomes bearing *single* genes, so that when a sperm fertilizes an egg and the genetic packages from each parent come together, the fusion results again in twenty-three *pairs* of chromosomes.

The genes also pair off once more, but in a new alignment to form an entirely new blueprint for a new and different person.

As the foetus is formed, these genes control factors like hair colour, hair type, eye colour, eye shape, nose shape, blood type, height and, indeed, every single characteristic.

It would be impossible (and far too complicated), even to try and follow the chain-gangs of worker genes as they direct, organize and specialize from the one original cell to the twenty-six trillion cells which go to make up a newborn baby. But each time the cells divide to form new ones, into them go exact replicas of all the chromosomes and all the genes. Many have work to do in every cell, but others only go into action if they are in a cell where their special craft is needed, making pigment for instance or perhaps forming bone or transmitting messages.

But one set of instructions is absolutely fundamental and this must be followed, because it is the one that determines sex and so for a woman initiates the oestrogen story.

Among the twenty-three pairs of chromosomes carried in every cell, there is one special pair of sex chromosomes. In women these are both of one type called X, and so the pair together form an XX combination. In men, however, there are two kinds, the familiar X type and a smaller Y type, giving an XY chromosome pair.

In the egg and the sperm, as we have seen, the pairs of chromosomes are split up. In the egg the sex chromosome must always be an X type, because this is the only sort a woman possesses. But among male sperm, some carry X type and some Y type in equal proportions.

So it is easy to see that it is the father, by the chance donation of either an X or Y sperm, who determines the sex of the baby. If a Y sperm wins the procreation race to penetrate and fertilize the female egg, which already contains its own X chromosome, this XY pair of chromosomes will produce a boy. If an X-bearing sperm is the first to reach the egg, the XX constitution makes a girl.

Despite this, to begin with and for some three months after conception, everyone is actually bisexual, equipped with the rudimentary organs and ducts for both sexes and capable of development in either direction. Only during, the fourth month of life in the womb, does nature's computer switch the foetus along a single-sex road. Programmed by an XY chromosome it commands the male organs and ducts to develop, leaving the female counterparts in their rudimentary state. Programmed by an XX chromosome, it triggers development of the female organs, leaving the male structure untouched. But once this sexual differentiation is begun, the sex hormones secreted by the growing testes or ovaries take over, and continue to govern the direction of development both before birth, and again later during puberty.

It is interesting that adults still retain some reminders of these bisexual beginnings. A man has clearly formed but non-functioning nipples, and a woman the clitoris, which is really the undeveloped penis.

One of the most fascinating bits of information, which modern knowledge has revealed and which must delight feminists, is that, quite contrary to Biblical mythology, it is the female which is the basic sex. It is now known that left to itself every foetus would turn toward the female. Only the powerful and continuous intervention of the male sex hormones, the androgens, effect the differentiation which results in a boy. So the legend of Lilith is after all more appropriate than that of Adam.

A male gynaecologist commenting on this, pointed out that rather less delightfully for Women's Lib, the female can be regarded as the neuter sex and the male as the positive and more advanced differentiation!

Whichever way you care to look at it, although the prototype female is already the basic sex, oestrogen must be present and in the right quantities, to ensure this female foetus developing fully and correctly.

In fact the balance between male and female hormones is crucial, both before birth and throughout life, and this fact too is related to continuing bisexual potential. Everyone produces some hormones of the other sex. Men produce small amounts of oestrogen and women secrete small amounts of androgens. So if at any time there is failure to produce enough of the right sex hormones to maintain the balance in the proper direction, there can be a tilt toward the opposite sex.

The foetus is particularly vulnerable in this respect. Too

much oestrogen reaching a male foetus can result in feminiza-
tion, and equally too much androgen reaching the female
foetus can mean a girl-baby being born with masculine traits,
maybe even an enlarged clitoris, which in the past could
sometimes tragically lead to wrong assignment of sex.

Fortunately such sexual ambiguity is rare, but the fact that
it can occur and the reasons for it, do serve to emphasize the
power and importance of the sex hormones.

The fate of the male castrate throughout history offers
another striking illustration. Deprived, either deliberately or
through accident, of his normal supply of male hormones
before puberty, the boy always retains a high voice, develops
female-pattern body hair and has no beard growth.

Hormonal imbalance sometimes shows up clearly for the
first time at puberty, with a girl failing to show the usual bud-
ding breasts or menstruation; or with a boy failing to develop
facial hair and deepening voice. Fortunately today, modern
endocrine knowledge provides the answer to such lack of
development or to late maturation. Appropriate hormone treatment is given, and maintained if necessary, to correct the situation.

The menopause on occasions offers a similar example of
hormone imbalance at work. In some older women declining
oestrogen levels can tilt the balance so far toward the male,
that growth of facial hair is triggered and occasionally the
voice too is affected becoming low and gruff. A very charming
woman, whom I know well, found her voice affected in this way
after the menopause. She told me, 'It led to ridiculous confusion on the telephone. I was always being mistaken for my
husband or my son. I tried to keep a sense of humour, but it
was pretty shattering to be called Mr.'

Hormone Replacement Therapy quickly corrected the voice
problem for her. It can often also help with facial hair. But it
is simpler, if possible, to *prevent* the imbalance and hirsuteness.
Once the hair follicles have been triggered, it is not always
easy to stop the growth.

All this could seem to present a daunting picture, but it
should be remembered that, for most people, nature's computer
works well and the direction of sexual development and drive is
clear-cut and normal.

For a girl, oestrogen continues to play a vital role. At first the young ovaries only produce very minute quantities, but such small traces can still be clearly detected in the urine, and it is believed that even these low levels of oestrogen may account for the more rapid skeletal maturation, and the earlier onset of puberty, in girls, as opposed to boys.

It is around the age of eleven or twelve, sometimes a little earlier, that the master gland, the pituitary, signals the ovaries to step up oestrogen production. Just as it once influenced the foetus toward the female, so now the increased oestrogen begins to resculpture the girl into the woman. The flat-chested tomboy is transformed, as breasts and nipples develop, the pelvis widens and fat appears on the hips to give rounded adult contours.

These higher levels of circulating oestrogen also stimulate the growth of external and internal genitalia, secretion of vaginal mucus, pigmentation of the nipples and development of pubic and axillary hair.

But the final act in the drama, the truly sensational transformation scene, comes with the release of the first egg and the establishment of regular menstruation and ovulation. This cyclic monthly rhythm, which becomes so much part of female life, is controlled by a hormonal ebb and flow, involving a complex feed-back mechanism between the pituitary and the ovaries.

First the pituitary gland secretes minute quantities of another hormone, known as FSH (follicle stimulating hormone) a name which describes exactly what it does. Less than a millionth of an ounce a day is sufficient to awaken a few dormant egg cells, and set off a dazzling chain of events.

Around each awakened egg there forms a fluid-filled follicle (a tiny protective sac). Usually only one follicle grows and expands sufficiently to push its way through and actually appear on the surface of the ovary, as a sort of bubble. Where, on rare occasions, two follicles do succeed in doing this, the potential situation exists for conception of non-identical twins.

The growing follicle now secretes more oestrogen to add to that already at work, instructing the uterus (womb) to prepare a thick lining, where any fertilized egg may become implanted and nourished.

The rising levels of oestrogen are sensed by the pituitary and another command goes out. This time yet another hormone, LH (luteinizing hormone), joints FSH and, about mid-cycle, their combined efforts cause the follicle to rupture releasing the egg, which is swept down through the Fallopian tubes into the uterus.

When the egg breaks out of its follicle it makes quite a tear in the membrane covering the ovary, and some women can actually feel this happen and experience a short sharp pain. When this ovulation occurs there is also a slight rise in temperature. This can be detected and used by women, both in trying to achieve conception or in trying to avoid it, as obviously it signals the time when there is the best chance of bringing the sperm and egg together.

But meanwhile a remarkable process is going on. The scar tissue on the ovary turns into a yellow gland, called the corpus luteum, and this sets about producing that other important female hormone, progesterone. Again the name indicates its main function, for it means pro-gestation or pro-pregnancy, and progesterone is known as the pregnancy hormone. Its main job is to preserve and modify the uterine lining ready for the fertilized egg.

However, if no conception takes place, after about twelve to fourteen days, the corpus luteum dies and the supply of progesterone is shut off, while the level of oestrogen also drops. These changes tell the waiting uterus that no baby has been conceived this time, and so the lining that has been built up is allowed to flow away, and with it the unfertilized egg. This is menstruation.

Needless to say, a mechanism so strong, sturdy and persistent that, against all odds, it has ensured the survival of the human race through a million hostile years, does not give up or become easily discouraged. The hormonal chain of command simply resumes operation – other follicles form – oestrogen levels are raised and the whole process begins again.

From all this the central role of oestrogen in the life of women is clear, but it goes far beyond this direct control of reproduction. Oestrogen is also carried in the bloodstream to affect every cell in the body. Protein, the basic substance of all cells, contains nitrogen as one of its most important ingredients, and oestrogen has the invaluable ability of enabling cells to assimilate nitrogen from food more effectively and utilize it more efficiently.

The importance of oestrogen in maintaining what is termed a 'positive nitrogen balance' is recognized in medicine. Oestrogen is administered on occasions to quite young girls, even at the risk of temporary premature maturation, and equally to quite old ladies, to help build up the nitrogen balance and ensure better cell nutrition in certain illnesses.

So the very presence of oestrogen in our bodies helps to ensure healthy cells, and this means, in particular, strong bones and tissues, giving good muscle tone, firm breasts, supple joints, clear skin and shining hair. Perhaps the clearest example of the special bloom oestrogen can give is seen in many women during healthy pregnancies, when oestrogen levels are at their highest.

Some strange and unexpected minor effects of oestrogen have recently been discovered through the work of a well-known, British zoologist, Professor John Ebling. He has shown that normal women are far more sensitive to the scent of musk, the smell derived from male animals such as the civet, than men are. As this is the basis of most classical perfumes, the sexy scents women use to turn men on probably work indirectly by turning on the women themselves first. The smell has to be a thousand times stronger for a man to notice it than a woman. But if a woman has her ovaries removed, then the scent of musk becomes as faint for her as for a man. Given Hormone Replacement, however, the scent once again becomes vivid and exciting.

Although many of the effects of oestrogen appear to be similarly concerned with keeping women sexually attractive and sexually responsive (both states clearly favoured by evolutionary forces during the fertile years), it does also carry out even more vital tasks, not so readily apparent.

There is, for example, the very specific job which oestrogen, and only oestrogen, can do in maturing the cells of the vagina, keeping it supple, elastic, free from infection and ready for both intercourse and childbirth. This forms the basis for the very simple test, which is described in a later chapter, which can establish the oestrogen level for any woman at any given time.

In much the same way oestrogen is now known to be involved in keeping arteries elastic, so helping to protect women
against arterial disease. And its positive effect in maintaining
muscle tone also protects against prolapse and against bladder
and urinary problems.

But the effects of the sex hormones can go beyond the entirely physical into the psychological. Because of the feed-back
mechanism and the strong link with the pituitary gland,
oestrogen and progesterone levels affect emotional stability. It
is no coincidence that many women feel depressed, nervy, and
irritable just before menstruation, when hormone levels drop.
The same kind of reaction can occur at the menopause, and
again it is no coincidence that both then and just before menstruation, women have more accidents and commit more
crimes. Both this 'pre-menstrual tension', as it is called, and
the menopause, respond to hormone treatment.

In many ways oestrogen has a place in the life of a woman
rather like that of love itself. She is born with both, and
both assume their greatest importance in her fertile years.
What is more she may take them both very much for granted,
and only fully realizes their value when they are gone.

One eminent British gynaecologist, who was strongly opposed
to Hormone Replacement Therapy, told me, 'What a woman
needs at the menopause is not oestrogen but a good husband.'
It is obviously even better to have both. But while love and
husbands cannot be had on prescription or be easily replaced,
fortunately, today, oestrogen can.

3. Oestrogen deficiency – the long and the short of it

For most women the first sign of the onset of the menopause is a change in the pattern of menstruation. If this has been regular, it becomes less so; if it has been irregular, it becomes more so; for other women the periods may just come at increasingly longer intervals, be unusually heavy, or simply become scanty and perhaps dark in colour, until, eventually, they cease altogether. The whole process may last for as long as five years, though in a few cases menstruation just ceases abruptly with no prior warning.

This abrupt cessation happens, of course, in the case also of women who undergo an operation involving removal of ovaries or where ovaries are destroyed by irradiation. Both a surgical menopause or radium menopause bring a rapid fall in oestrogen levels, and often the swift onset of symptoms.

Not all women suffer all symptoms, and this is really just as well, for there are some twenty-one recognized symptoms associated with the menopause. There are even some women who seem to sail through the change of life with no problems at all. These are the fortunate ones, estimated at around 15%, whose adrenal glands seem able to step up oestrogen sufficiently to compensate for the failing ovaries. Eventually, however, though at a much later stage, oestrogen deficiency usually catches up with them too, though it may not by then produce any overt symptoms.

For the rest, the other 85%, symptoms most common at the onset of the menopause are fatigue, headaches, irritability, palpitations, dizziness and, to a lesser degree, depression. These mark the beginning of the disturbances arising from hormone imbalance.

Hot flushes (or flashes, which somehow sounds more dramatic), night sweats, and pains in the joints and muscles usually come rather later, in the early post-menopause, that is soon after ovarian function and menstruation have ceased.

Another very strange symptom which many women have mentioned to me is officially called 'formication' – a word which demands rather careful spelling! It is the medical term for the peculiar crawling sensation near the body surface, which one American woman described to me as feeling like 'an army of ants walking about under your skin'.

An interesting research, so far as I can find the first of its kind, was recently carried out by the International Health Foundation, to study the attitude of women toward the menopause in five European countries – a sort of menopausal Common Market. The study was based on personal interviews with two thousand women, all between the ages of forty-six and fifty-five, from Belgium, France, Great Britain, Italy and West Germany.

Questions were asked about memories of their mothers' experiences, about their own experiences, and about their attitudes toward the menopause and life after it. They were also asked how much they knew about medical treatment available, and if they had sought such help.

Some fascinating cultural differences emerged, with British women, in proverbial stiff upper lip tradition, taking the most optimistic and stoical view. The women of Belgium and Italy were the most gloomy, and in particular, twice as many of them thought the menopause marked not only the start of old age, but the end of their attractiveness to men.

The symptoms most commonly experienced throughout the menopause proved to be: 55% flushes, 43% tiredness, 41% nervousness, 39% sweating, 38% headaches, 32% insomnia, 30% depression, 29% irritability, 25% joint and muscle pains, 24% dizziness, 24% palpitations and 22% pins and needles, which is perhaps similar to the tingling, crawling sensation.

Over all, it is interesting to find that although 86% said they suffered during the menopause, only 52% had actually sought medical help. Obviously intensity and duration of symptoms must partly determine this, but it also seems likely that the numbers seeking help are related to the numbers knowing that such help existed. Only 53% knew there was any medical treatment to lessen the problems of the menopause, and British women were particularly ill-informed. Only 36% of British women had heard of any medical treatment as against

71% in West Germany, 57% in Belgium, 54% in France and 47% in Italy.

Among those who knew treatment existed, the West Germans were the best informed. 66% of those who knew also actually mentioned oestrogen replacement or hormone treatment, while the comparative figures for those who had heard of HRT in the other countries were 41% in Italy, 40% in France, 22% in Belgium and Great Britain. No comparable figures are available for the USA, but a snap survey done for this book confirmed a similar percentage of women experiencing menopause problems, but a far greater percentage aware of the possibilities of what they simply termed 'hormones' or 'oestrogen'.

Earlier this century, in fact up to the second world war, the average age for final menstruation was around forty-eight. Recent surveys, including one among over six thousand women in Holland, have shown this age has risen now to over fifty-one. With earlier puberty this means the fertile life of women is extending at both ends, perhaps to match the longer life expectancy. The Dutch survey also found that while 23% of women aged forty-one were already starting to experience irregular menstruation, approximately half of the women aged forty-six, forty-seven and forty-eight still reported their menstrual cycles as regular. After that, however, the percentage with regular cycles decreases rapidly.

Although research and surveys reveal a general basic pattern in both onset and symptoms, the menopause experience for each woman remains intensely individual. Not only does severity, duration and number of symptoms vary for everyone, but so does reaction, attitude and situation.

The hot flushes, which one woman may tolerate well within home and family, can be quite intolerable and embarrassing to a woman holding down a job, which involves contact with the public or with male colleagues.

Both the International Health Foundation survey and my own enquiries confirm that most women worry as much about the psychological aspects of the change of life as about the physical. It is worrying to be subject to sweating and head-aches, to put on weight or lose that once firm figure, but it is just as worrying to lose one's memory, lack confidence or become subject to confusion and depression.

B

Barbara Simpson, Deputy Head of a large mixed Comprehensive School in England, wrote to me after my series of articles first appeared, and her case not only illustrates this point, but emphasizes the difference between the American and the British scene. She wrote,

. . . I was working in America and was put on Premarin (natural oestrogen) immediately following a hysterectomy over there three years ago. I was absolutely fine, physically and mentally until I came back to England, where to my horror my own doctor insisted I come off the therapy. He gradually cut down the dosage until I was off it completely. I soon became aware of hot flushes and more gradually of growing confusion, lack of memory and lack of confidence. In my job, working with male colleagues and boys of up to sixteen, the flushes which made me go red and hot were very embarrassing. But even worse was the growing inability to concentrate. You can imagine in this job, I have to keep right on top. Needless to say I have been back to my doctor but he adamantly refuses to renew the prescription and I am becoming desperate. Now I know from your article that the therapy is obtainable in this country, I am determined to change my doctor . . .

Barbara Simpson was an intelligent and determined woman and once she knew Hormone Replacement *was* available she obtained it, and reported back to me that it worked like a miracle and she was again thriving. She went privately to a gynaecologist, and later also changed to another group practice of GP's, where the doctors, although not too familiar with the treatment, were at least prepared to carry out the gynaecologist's recommended regime.

One of the most distressing physical symptoms of oestrogen deficiency, which women experience very often after surgical removal of ovaries and also in the natural post-menopause, is vaginal dryness and atrophy, often so severe that intercourse becomes painful or impossible.

It seems possible that the medical profession underestimates this problem, because so many letters I receive mention it and also stress the fact that the writers are too shy to discuss it with their doctors. Once they know effective treatment exists, they usually pluck up courage to mention the problem, but even then unfortunately there is no guarantee that oestrogen replacement will be prescribed.

Because this is one of the symptoms most closely and directly linked to lack of oestrogen, and one which is effectively and swiftly relieved, either by oestrogen tablets taken orally, or by oestrogen cream applied locally, it is particularly tragic that it should so often go untreated. The lubricants and vaginal jellies sometimes prescribed are, at best, only palliatives, and do nothing to remove the basic cause. Oestrogen replacement can relieve the condition within weeks. Replacement Therapy started early enough, of course, prevents it ever happening.

Dozens of women wrote desperate and moving letters about this problem, many of them showing clearly how this meno-pause symptom in particular casts a long shadow, beyond the woman herself, to darken and endanger both marriage and family stability.

A typical letter from a fifty-year-old English woman ran,

Your articles on Hormone Replacement Therapy brought me the first hope in five years. I began the menopause five years ago. Since then I have suffered not only the usual physical symptoms, particularly back-aches and night sweats, but also insomnia, confusion and depression.

My doctor says it is 'natural' and 'just my age', and gives me pain-killers for my back and Librium for what he calls my 'bad nerves'. All his treatment does is make me more tired, so that I get more irritable.

I love my husband and two sons very much but I know I have become a misery to live with.

I used to enjoy a normal sex life, but now it is something I dread because it is so painful. Recently I bought twin beds, pretending it was because I was so restless, but really it was to avoid him wanting me.

I am truly afraid for my marriage if this goes on, and my doctor refuses even to read your article or consider giving me oestrogen. I do a part-time job and would be happy to pay for the treatment if it would help me get back to normal. My family can't understand my misery.

This woman finally received help, and took the trouble to write me happily a few months later to say she had been to a doctor in London who specialized in Hormone Replacement. After a test to establish that her oestrogen levels were low, he had put her on natural oestrogen. Within weeks 'life became worth living again', to use her own phrase.

Depression is a symptom which many women complain about in their letters. By no means all middle-aged depression is hormone-based, and this will be discussed in greater detail in later chapters. But some of it is essentially rooted in the disturbances which oestrogen deprivation causes in the autonomic nervous system. The case of Mrs Joan Williams illustrates this well. Aged fifty-five when I met her, she had been struggling since the end of menstruation five years before with terrible night sweats and palpitations. She told me,

It was so bad that I could only sleep if I was drugged. All my doctor would do, and it was a woman doctor, was give me Librium and Valium to help me sleep. She said she couldn't do anything else, it was 'just my age'. The worst part was the awful depression and lack of confidence. I got that I couldn't go out or talk to anyone; I just wanted to curl up and sleep the day away . . .

I did fight against it. I struggled at first to look after my home and go out to work, because I didn't want to give in. My husband didn't understand, and all he would say was 'Pull yourself together'. In the end I just had to give up the job. I felt so ill and so desperate that I really thought I was going to die.

Then I read your articles in *The Birmingham Mail*. I'd got a bit of money saved from my job and my husband said he'd give anything to get me back to normal, so we decided I should go privately to a gynaecologist. It wasn't after all very expensive, but I can't tell you what it was like to have someone to talk to who really understood. You see I really thought I might be going off my head. In fact I'd even asked my own doctor if I could pay to go and see a psychiatrist. Then that gynaecologist explained it all, and told me other women felt the same way. She gave me a thorough examination, checked my oestrogen level and put me on to Replacement Therapy. Within two weeks the physical symptoms had gone completely. After all these years I could hardly believe it.

Quite soon the depression lifted and then I began to get my confidence back. Now I am planning to start a job again. My husband is amazed to see me taking an interest in my hair again and in my looks. He understands now that it was a physical thing, not just something in my mind.

So far all the symptoms discussed, both mental and physical, have been the sort which show up clearly and quickly, and of which a woman is only too well aware herself. But there are others, unseen and insidious, which in the long-term can cause far more serious problems.

4. Long-term protection

Symptoms which can be seen and felt can be dealt with in one way or another. A woman suffering from lack of energy or head-aches can either adapt by taking more rest or, if this does not work, seek help from her doctor. She is aware of what is happening.

Far more frightening and disconcerting is the stealthy and secret onset of the condition known as osteoporosis, which involves steady loss of healthy bone over the years, without the victim even being aware of the process in the early stages. The first warning that a woman may have that her bones have become porous and brittle can be the onset of low back-pain in the late post-menopause. Over the years there may also be progressive loss of height and even in some cases the gradual appearance of the dreaded 'dowager's hump', which disfigures so many old ladies.

But the most common way in which osteoporosis shows up, and usually without any earlier pain to act as warning, is in the sudden fracture of wrist or thigh after quite a light fall.

It was the fact that women who had had their ovaries re-moved developed osteoporosis very early that first linked the disease to lack of sex hormones. Women develop it far more often than men and in addition they develop it far earlier than men, and this was thought to be related to the much later and slower decline of male sex hormones, which allowed their protective role to last longer. Osteoporosis is, in fact, four times more common in women than in men. If other corroborative evidence were needed, there was the dramatic rise in fractures of the wrist for women after the menopause. These were found to go up ten times, while in men there was only a very slight rise when they were almost eighty.

Not all menopausal women develop acute osteoporosis, but one figure, now thought to be on the low side, estimates 25% have it to some degree, and in all menopausal women there is a steep rise in bone resorption rates.

It is this rise in resorption and the consequent reduction in the amount of bony tissue that leads to osteoporosis. The overall bone loss in women between the ages of fifty and eighty can represent about 15% of the skeleton. Small wonder in the already lighter bones of women this leads to fractures of wrist and thigh and crush fractures of the vertebrae. Of the estimated six million suffering from this disease in the States, five million are post-menopausal women.

In Great Britain it has been estimated that about five thousand hospital beds are constantly occupied by hip fracture cases, at the annual cost of well over ten million pounds.

There is a special sadness somehow in the knowledge that the old lady of eighty, who breaks her hip or wrist after only a slight fall, can blame it on the fact that her ovaries packed up some thirty years before, and no one did anything about it.

The newspapers are always carrying stories of such accidents. The British papers in 1971 reported the Duchess of Windsor breaking her hip, and the year before that it was Lady Churchill. The big names make the headlines, but in America alone more than a million women of forty-five and over fracture hips and other bones each year, and two-thirds of these cases are due to osteoporosis.

Of course the real test of the direct link with oestrogen deficiency lies in the effectiveness of oestrogen in treating osteoporosis and in preventing bone resorption.

A great deal of work has been done in this area. In San Francisco, where he is Professor of Medicine and Chief of both the Endocrine and Bone Clinics at the University of California Medical Center, I talked to Dr Gilbert Gordan. A world expert on osteoporosis, he is among the many doctors now using oestrogen treatment to combat the condition. He told me, 'We find it is the single most effective treatment. We use natural oestrogen, given cyclically, and in the large series of women treated over many years, a fracture has never been seen once the therapy has been properly instituted and maintained.'

Given early enough, Dr Gordan claims oestrogen replacement therapy prevents osteoporosis ever happening, but given belatedly after it has set in, he admits it can only arrest but not reverse the condition, though even then it gets rid of the pain and prevents further fractures.[1]

As an example of the fact that it is never too late, Polly Cartland, the remarkable ninety-seven-year-old mother of British romantic novelist, Barbara Cartland, and grandmother of the Countess of Dartmouth, was herself put on oestrogen after breaking a hip in her ninety-sixth year. Barbara Cartland told me, 'I went on natural oestrogen myself after a hysterectomy recently and felt just wonderful on it. My daughter who is in the mid-forties has gone on to it as preventative medicine, and now finally my mother has been put on it by her doctor to protect against risk of further fracture. So that is the three generations, and all thriving on it.'

Until recently British medicine has remained largely unconvinced about the effectiveness of oestrogen therapy in treating osteoporosis, but reports of new British research have now been published which strongly confirm the American claims.

At the Mineral Metabolism Unit at the Leeds General Infirmary, Dr Christopher Nordin and Dr J. Gallagher have determined the actual bone loss in women, both after normal menopause and after surgical menopause following removal of ovaries. They did this by checking the amounts of calcium excreted in the urine. The tests were carried out in the morning, after over-night fasting, to eliminate any of the calcium coming from food. Figures showed a dramatic rise in bone resorption rates for all these women, paralleling the already known tenfold rise in wrist fracture rates in post-menopausal women.[2]

Similar results were obtained in Glasgow by Dr J. M. Aitken and a team, who this time measured actual decrease in bone density by a new and accurate scanning method.[3]

Significantly in both studies, administration of oestrogen was found to bring resorption rates quickly back to premenopausal levels. Dr Nordin told me, 'Our work suggests that some 50% of menopausal women require replacement therapy. Without it the skeletal loss after the menopause can be as much as 2% a year.'

The Mineral Metabolism Unit at Leeds has also gone some way toward suggesting the mechanism at work. It had already been established that oestrogen appeared to block resorption of bone rather than actually induce production of new bone. The team at Leeds carried out experiments which suggest that oestrogen blocks the action of another hormone, parathyroid (PTH), which releases both calcium and phosphate from the bone.

The idea that the oestrogen might work in this way, to preserve a positive calcium balance and healthy bones, was indicated by the excessive bone loss seen in post-menopausal women with over-active parathyroid glands and excess parathyroid secretion.

Although there can be other contributory factors at work in the development of osteoporosis, such as inadequate mineral intake, poor mineral absorption and lack of physical activity, oestrogen deficiency is being increasingly recognized as the fundamental cause in women. More and more doctors are joining Dr Gordan in using long-term oestrogen replacement as preventative medicine against the onset of the disease, and also in treating it, where it already exists, with a combination of oestrogen therapy, increased calcium intake, adequate vitamin D and, where possible, increased exercise. Osteoporosis is accepted now as pathological dysfunction, and not an inevitable and untreatable part of ageing.

Quite as important as the protection oestrogen appears to afford against osteoporosis, is the protection it also seems to offer against cardiac trouble.

It is an accepted fact, of course, that during their reproductive years, when oestrogen levels are high, women rarely have heart attacks. The records show young men under forty are at least twenty times more prone than women of comparable age to this trouble.[5]

Yet, after the menopause when oestrogen production drops, women rapidly lose this built-in advantage. In the forty–forty-nine-year age group the ratio drops steeply to only three to one, and in the fifty–fifty-nine-year age group, it is down to two to one.

The blood fat most closely associated with a predisposition to heart attacks is cholesterol. Clinical studies have shown high cholesterol levels in men appear to be related to development of coronary artery disease, especially in the younger age groups.

Many doctors have believed for a long time that lack of oestrogen could be, in part, responsible for the increased levels of cholesterol in the blood, and certainly checks done on women after HRT has been instituted have shown a drop in cholesterol.[6]

Studies have also shown the blood cholesterol levels of young women are not only lower in general than those of young men, but are at their very lowest in each individual woman at mid-cycle when oestrogen levels are highest.

Conversely, women who have had ovaries removed and so have little oestrogen, show evidence of higher blood cholesterol compared to control groups of women of comparable age. They have also been shown to be more prone to heart disease.[7]

In one study of 102 women who had had ovaries removed, compared with 112 women of similar age who had only had the womb removed, it was found ten years after surgery that nineteen of the women without ovaries had experienced cardio-vascular disorders, as against only five in the other group. A further follow-up two years later, showed another seven with heart trouble in the castrated patients, but no more in the control group.

So it is becoming widely accepted in medicine now that the oestrogen in a woman's body helps to protect her against heart diseases, particularly arteriosclerosis which involves thickening and roughening of the normally smooth lining of the coronary arteries. Figures indicate that women whose ovaries are re-moved before the menopause are four times as likely to run into this sort of trouble as women who retain their ovaries.[8] Autop-sies have shown a 10%–45% greater occurrence of severe arteriosclerosis. For this reason, as well as to delay vaginal atrophy, surgeons where possible now prefer to leave one ovary or even part of an ovary.

But increasing evidence of the protective action of the body's own oestrogen is not the same as proving that *administered* oestrogen will do exactly the same thing, and a great deal of work is going on both in the USA and in Great Britain to try and determine this. The study already mentioned did actually throw up some hopeful evidence. Among the women without ovaries, just a small number were treated with oestrogen therapy, and in their cases the rate of cardio-vascular compli-cations was almost as low as in the controls.

Work has also been done to see if oestrogens will protect men with coronary histories against further heart trouble. The results are not conclusive though in one study where the dosage of oestrogen was too low to actually reduce the level of blood fats considered harmful, there was nevertheless a definite improvement in the survival rate and in another group the death rate was 50% less than for a control group of patients not receiving oestrogen. Unfortunately men treated with oestrogen often face unpleasant side effects, including breast enlargement, diminished libido and impotence.

In the past much of the research on this subject has been done with men, but currently two long-range studies of women are under way at a hospital in Massachusetts. They are designed to discover if oestrogen therapy can delay or prevent arteriosclerosis after the menopause, and also to determine its value in preventing further complications and prolonging life for women who have already suffered coronary attacks. Present evidence certainly suggests that oestrogen therapy should be seriously considered as preventive medicine against heart disease, and particularly for women who might be considered at high risk, such as heavy smokers or women with mounting blood pressure, obesity, high cholesterol, impaired thyroid or a family history of coronary disease or diabetes.[9]

Diabetes is another area where a lot of research is going on to try and determine if administered oestrogen works in the same way as the body's own oestrogen.

Again observation has shown that glucose tolerance declines with age and experiments have been carried out to see if this could be associated with loss of oestrogen and progesterone at the menopause.

At the Department of Biological Science at the University of Aston in Birmingham, England, a team of scientists under Professor A. J. Matty and Dr C. J. Bailey have not only proved that rats, whose ovaries have been removed, have impaired glucose tolerance, but have shown that injections of progesterone and of oestrogen both improved this again, giving higher blood insulin and lower blood sugar than in untreated controls. This, together with work on pancreas cells in vitro, both suggest that the hormones do promote secretion of insulin.[10]

It is still a big step to extrapolate from rats to humans, and much more work must be done. Meanwhile it would be interesting to discover if women developing diabetes include a high proportion who have had an early removal of ovaries, and also if among women on long-term HRT, there is a lower incidence of this disease.

Other long-term protection claimed for Hormone Replacement Therapy and increasingly widely used in Geriatric care, is preservation of muscle tone in the area of the bladder to prevent one of the most dreaded symptoms of old age, incontinence.[11]

Among elderly ladies on both sides of the Atlantic, oestrogen therapy has been found to have beneficial results in this respect and in relation to uterine prolapse. In some cases it has restored tone so well to pelvic supporting structures that the need for surgery has been obviated, and indeed some doctors now believe HRT is more effective than surgery where the degree of prolapse is not too severe.

Where controlled trials were carried out, it was also found that those elderly patients receiving oestrogen therapy also became less apathetic and more interested in life than untreated patients.[12]

Very similar results were reported by a British doctor, John Maddison. He became convinced of the value of HRT when running a Geriatric Centre at Teddington, and he carried out trials over a fifteen-year period. He told me, 'We observed the clinical state of some two thousand old people, taking regular checks for height, strength of hand-grip, mental ability and so on. Among the women half were given oestrogen and half were not. Those on oestrogen replacement showed no loss of height, while among the others there was up to two inches loss over the period due to osteoporosis. The ones on oestrogen also kept happier and more alert.'

All the forms of long-term protection so far mentioned in connection with oestrogen replacement have their special importance. Osteoporosis can cripple, heart disease can kill and even the common and unheroic incontinence can make life a misery both for the elderly victim, who is often miserably sensitive and shamed, and for relatives or nurses who have to cope with it.

But there is one form of possible long-term protection not yet mentioned, which is so important that it warrants separate consideration. And so in the next chapter we shall be looking at the growing evidence that long-term oestrogen therapy protects against cancer.

5. Protection against cancer?

In science and in medicine one discovery leads to another; one set of observations suggests a further line of enquiry. It was in this way that Dr Gordan in San Francisco made the most startling discovery of all about the possible protective role of oestrogen. In the follow-up of women on long-term cyclic oestrogen treatment for osteoporosis, he found that there was an unexpected and significant reduction in the incidence of all forms of cancer.[1]

Similar reports began to come in from other independent studies, and that respected British medical paper, *The Lancet*, drew attention to these findings in January, 1971. Four studies were quoted involving 1130 female patients, treated with cyclic estrogen for between five and seventeen years. The normal expected number of cancers should have been seventy-six. There were two.

In another study of 1422 women, made by Professor John Bakke, some ninety-six cases of cancer would have been expected to show up, and there were only five. A more recent study of 292 patients on long-term oestrogen revealed no cases of breast cancer at all, when statistically there should have been sixteen.[2]

But the firmest, most up to date and most authenticated figures come from an intriguing retrospective study recently reported in the *American Annals of Surgery*. Two doctors, John Burch and Benjamin Byrd, working at Vanderbilt University School of Medicine, Nashville, Tennessee, carried out a 100% follow-up of 713 patients, ranging in age from twenty-seven to eighty-five. All these women had undergone hysterectomy, their operations occurring between 1948 and 1967, and all had received continuous oestrogen replacement therapy from shortly after surgery onwards. This meant that all the patients had been on therapy for nine years or more, with some on oestrogen for over twenty years.[3]

The study set out in particular to look at three things, the incidence of breast cancer, the incidence of all forms of cancer; and the general mortality rate.

The results of the study were so startling that they were subjected to the most careful scrutiny available both medically and statistically. No criticism could be found, and in all cases when drawing statistical comparisons, figures had already been corrected to allow for the hysterectomies having eliminated uterine cancer risk.

Briefly the survey showed that although the number of breast cancers in the group were comparable to that which would be anticipated in any group of women of the same ages, in the group treated with oestrogen *they came ten years later.*

The incidence of *all* cancers showed a steady decline, with only *one-third of the anticipated incidence in treated women of forty and over.* But most dramatic of all, after the age of forty-five, the mortality rate in the treated women dropped to *only half the mortality expected in women of comparable ages.*

The postponement of the onset of breast cancer by ten years has special significance, because it goes beyond just winning an extra decade free of the disease. The later cancer strikes, the slower as a rule is its rate of progression, and the better the chance of a cure.

In 1974 I went to Nashville, Tennessee, to visit doctors Burch and Byrd.

Dr Burch explained to me how they had come to undertake the survey, 'It was a casual conversation in the scrub room one morning. Dr Byrd had a patient with mammary cancer in one room and I had one in another, and he asked the question: "Did I think oestrogen treatment had anything to do with it?" I said, "I don't believe so" and Dr Byrd said, "Well now, what do you do to back your belief up?" I told him I thought I had the cases to give the answer.'

It was from Dr Burch's extensive log of patients that the follow-up was done. Fortunately, in a comparatively small and stable community, it proved possible to trace every one. Dr Byrd described their reactions to the results. 'We were shocked,' he told me. 'Not so much at the mammary cancer figures, because from our experience we had felt oestrogen therapy produced no significant rise in incidence, but we had not appreciated the delaying effect. Then the low incidence of

all forms of cancer and the decrease in mortality were staggering. Where seventy-six cancers would be expected only
thirty-five occurred. There were only nine deaths from heart
attacks where twenty-one would be expected and a total of
forty deaths in the group where ninety-four would be expected.

In fact the results were so staggering that the two men told
me it was not easy to decide whether to publish them. They
first subjected the survey and the conclusions to the most
rigorous examination by independent experts. Dr Byrd
explained, 'We were worried about turning loose this sort of
information and the position we would have to take up. But
when the figures and conclusions were so completely vindicated
by outside examination, we decided it would be as wrong to keep
evidence of benefit back as to suppress any evidence of risk.'

Other benefits which the survey revealed were a significant
decrease in the number of wrist fractures – only two-thirds the
expected number. Also 477 out of 550 women in the survey,
who were personally asked how they felt on oestrogen therapy,
insisted that they felt better than before treatment. While
Dr Byrd acknowledged that this was a subjective judgement,
he added, 'All the same it is obvious these women do feel good.
They look good. Their skin is clear. They seem to be staying
young.'

It was the low incidence of cancer combined with the low
incidence of heart disease which accounted for the tremendous
50% drop in mortality rates in the over-forty-five age group.
So, the Nashville survey also produced support for the claim
that oestrogen therapy gives long-term protection against
arterial and heart disease.

A great deal more work will have to be done and far more
studies made, before anyone can claim that long-term cyclic
oestrogen positively protects against cancer. For one thing
cancer is a condition of undisciplined cell division, rather than
a single disease, and it almost certainly has many different
causes to which eventually must be found many different
answers. But so far at least the indications for oestrogen exerting
beneficial influence are strong.

As clinical and statistical evidence grows of the protective
role of oestrogen in regard to many forms of disease, more and
more research is directed toward finding out *how* it works.

One man, whose life-time study of the body defence mechanism throws light on the problem, is Professor Thomas Nicol. Professor of Anatomy at King's College, London, for thirty-one years, he now works at The Institute of Laryngology and Otology in London.

Professor Nicol told me, 'More than thirty years of research and thousands of experiments have provided convincing proof that oestrogen is the natural stimulant of the body's defences against infection, premature ageing and certain forms of cancer. It is the petrol that fuels the whole defence system.

'Our experiments have shown that oestrogen stimulates the white cells of the blood and increases their power to mop up invading organisms. This ability of oestrogen to activate the defence mechanism explains why men do not generally live as long as women, whose bodies consistently produce more oestrogen. It also explains why pregnant women, who have high oestrogen levels, are usually healthier and less liable to infection. Further it explains the fact that depression, fear and worry are able to lower resistance and damage the body's defences, almost certainly through a feed-back mechanism affecting hormone balance.[4]

'Fortunately the new technique of radioimmunoassay, which now enables us to measure hormone levels in the blood accurately, may make it possible to rectify the hormone imbalances which come with ageing. The essential problem now is to establish healthy norms, the base-line from which to work.'

This is very much the way in which ideally HRT should work, with the individual normal oestrogen level for each woman established before the onset of the menopause causes the levels to drop. Later chapters and case-histories explain this concept in more detail.

But meanwhile with the short-term advantages so clearly obvious, and the long-term protective role so strongly indicated, women are entitled to ask why medicine has been so reluctant to accept HRT? With hormone replacement already accepted and conventional treatment for other forms of hormone deficiency, for thyroid, adrenal and for diabetes, why has oestrogen deficiency at the menopause been felt to be different? What are the objections some doctors still raise when women ask them for oestrogen to help them through the menopause?

6. The medical controversy

Although some 80% of American gynaecologists are estimated to subscribe to the concept of Hormone Replacement Therapy at the menopause, this does not mean there is no opposition. Right from the first this has been highly controversial medicine, involving strong views and feelings.

In the States today there are still many who openly declare the idea of treating the menopause as a deficiency condition is dangerous nonsense, and others who content themselves with arguing that it is simply unnecessary and the benefits unproven.

In both America and Britain until very recently the hard-core resistance has come from the older family or country physician, who has often only vaguely heard about HRT. Many such doctors have confessed to me that they knew little about it, but they often added that they distrusted oestrogens on principle, and in any case felt women could get through the menopause quite well as their mothers had done, without such new-fangled notions.

Young doctors, as might be expected, were more interested and open-minded. Where they did not already know much about it, some, like my own doctor, took the trouble to read up on it, and once this was done they usually began to prescribe, only cautiously at first in severe cases of menopause problems, but later, gaining confidence with each success, they became converted to wider use.

In both countries the prevailing attitude in any one area tended to stem from the top, where the leading gynaecologists' known views exerted considerable influence. In one area in Britain, where at the time HRT was particularly hard to get, the leading gynaecologist told me flatly, 'I am horrified at the idea of looking at the menopause as a disease. This kind of thinking is for the birds and for those in private practice who have time on their hands, where, no doubt, it will prove a goldmine.'

Having gone on to condemn HRT as unnecessary in anything but very small doses to relieve really acute symptoms, I was amused at one final reservation. He added, 'I would say if a menopausal woman marries again, she should have oestrogen replacement as it keeps the vagina young.' Presumably women still on Mark 1 husbands and marriages can just struggle on with old vaginas!

In fairness I must add that this particular consultant, despite personal lack of enthusiasm for replacement therapy, still allowed a younger man in his Professorial Unit to set up a special clinic where the problems of the menopause and the role of HRT could be studied.

Clinics like this with planned programmes of HRT, and research backed by the facilities of large hospitals and combined with well-kept records, are the basis of many current studies which could well achieve the full and final breakthrough for replacement therapy at the menopause. Professor Jack Dewhurst, one of Britain's leading gynaecologists, is carrying out similar treatment and trials at his Menopausal Clinic at Chelsea Women's Hospital in London.

Professor Dewhurst told me, 'There is a need for further examination of possible wider usage of Hormone Replacement for at least some post-menopausal women, and it is for this that we have set up our clinic. The work done so far certainly confirms that symptoms, particularly hot flushes, and genital tract changes benefit enormously. It is a good deal less certain if headaches, palpitations and depression are directly dependent on hormones. There is a great deal of work still to be done.'[1]

Some of that work is being done at another similar clinic at Birmingham Women's Hospital, set up specially to evaluate HRT in the treatment of the menopause. Preliminary results presented at the 1974 20th British Congress of Obstetrics and Gynaecology in London, reported 100% control of hot flushes and also confirmed the protective role of oestrogen over the skeletal system. As well as improved calcium and cholesterol levels, a striking 27.8% reduction was observed in the level of an enzyme called alkaline phosphatase[2]. This enzyme normally rises steeply at the menopause, and the reduction suggests that HRT may have beneficial effects on liver function.

On the other hand it has been said there is some evidence

from other sources of oestrogen administration being associated with a higher incidence of gall-bladder diseases.

The *New England Journal of Medicine* for January 3, 1973, alerted readers to the findings of the Boston Collaborative Drug Surveillance programme. A study had been made of more than five thousand women, aged between forty-five and sixty-nine, admitted to hospital in the Massachusetts area. A comparison was made between those with gall-stones or inflammation of the gall-bladder and a control group of women admitted to hospital for other reasons. Treatment with oestrogens was two and a half times as common in the women with gall-bladder disease. But no similar evidence was found of any link between oestrogen treatment and either breast tumours or thrombotic disorders.

Weighing up evidence can be very much a matter of swings and roundabouts – the gall-bladder finding was new and adverse, but the reassuring findings on thrombosis and cancer risk offset this by helping to dismiss the two main fears connected with HRT.[3]

Invariably when I ask a doctor opposed to the use of HRT why he will not prescribe the treatment he mentions three things; the cancer risk; the thrombosis risk; and breakthrough bleeding. So let us look at each in turn.

In view of the statistical evidence we have already seen suggesting women on oestrogen therapy have a lower incidence of cancer, it is surprising to find how strongly the opposite view persists that oestrogens in some way may cause cancer. It is usually at family doctor level that I find this fear exists and it is all rather vague, just dark mutterings about a possible link and in some cases actual mention of what they called 'the stilbestrol scare'. Because this undoubtedly underlies most of the worry, it must be described and evaluated.

Stilbestrol is known as a synthetic oestrogen, but in fact it is a coal-tar derivative which cannot properly be described as an oestrogen at all, but which possesses oestrogenic properties – that is it performs some of the functions of an oestrogen. In particular it can help to prevent miscarriage and get rid of milk after pregnancy. It is cheap, effective and was, therefore, at one time widely used both for these purposes and to treat menopausal problems.

Back in the '30s, in the early days of cancer research and hormone research, which developed together, many substances were tried out for cancer-producing properties, and one of them was stilbestrol. Massive amounts were given to laboratory-bred mice and tumours were produced. As coal-tar derivatives are now known carcinogens this was not really too surprising, especially as the mice were a special cancer-prone strain and were fed half their own bodyweight of stilbestrol over a six-month period, which represents about a quarter of their normal life span. It has been estimated a woman would have to swallow about 150 lbs of oestrogen over half her lifetime to receive a comparable dose.[4]

Experiments done at the same time to produce similar tumours by feeding stilbestrol to mice, belonging to a strain in which spontaneous breast cancer seldom occurred in the females, entirely failed. In fact all further experiments since then, feeding oestrogens to mice, rats and even more relevantly to monkeys over a ten-year period, have all failed to reproduce any forms of cancer.[5]

But fears regarding stilbestrol were newly aroused in 1971, when reports were received from the New England area that some female offspring of women, treated with stilbestrol some twenty years previously to prevent miscarriage, had developed vaginal cancers after puberty. Thirteen young girls were involved in the early reports, aged between fifteen and twenty-two years, all with a form of vaginal cancer which is most uncommon and usually only occurs at a much older age. Investigation showed that in twelve out of the thirteen cases, the mothers had been treated with stilbestrol for threatened miscarriage from the first two months almost to term. Since then further cases have been uncovered and the latest report in the *American Journal of Obstetrics and Gynecology* for the 1st July 1974, mentioned an appalling total of 170 girls affected.[6]

It is important to emphasize that in no case did the mother herself develop any form of cancer, but it is clearly an example, and a terrible one, of the extreme vulnerability of the foetus to hormone influence, with puberty probably acting as a second hormone trigger.

A top American gynaecologist and endocrinologist with whom I discussed these tragedies explained, 'The stilbestrol clearly crossed the placental barrier and the foetal liver could not metabolize it. It is obviously different with natural oestrogen, because mothers have colossal amounts of this in their bodies during pregnancy and the foetus is unaffected.'

The lesson to be learned from this, of course, is that stilbestrol should never be used to treat a pregnant woman, and in fact with the wide choice of oestrogens now available there is little argument for it ever being used at all – it remains a coal-tar derivative, not a true oestrogen, and must be suspect.

Unfortunately, where busy doctors have no time or opportunity to study the low cancer record of long-term oestrogen replacement, they can easily project the sinister shadow hanging over stilbestrol onto other innocent oestrogens. Also in the minds of some doctors who fear a link between hormones and cancer, is the fact that some forms of breast cancer can be what is termed 'hormone dependent', that is, their cell growth is stimulated by hormones. In such cases at one time, it was not unusual for the ovaries to be removed in an attempt to slow down progress of the disease.

Stimulating the growth of an existing tumour is very different to *causing* it in the first place, but this distinction is not always sufficiently emphasized. In fact, this type of hormone-dependent cancer of the breast usually only occurs in *young* women, and when it does, they are advised against the contraceptive pill with its quota of synthetic oestrogen. They are extremely rare in older women, and a history of successfully treated breast cancer is by no means always a contra-indication for HRT at the menopause.

Just as experiments using heavy, long-term and continuous oestrogen stimulation entirely failed to induce breast cancer in monkeys, so also did they fail to produce uterine cancer. This is specially important because oestrogen given alone over a prolonged time without interruption can cause an abnormal build-up of the lining of the uterus. This condition, known as hyperplasia, can exist with or precede uterine cancer, so that again although oestrogen is not implicated as a *cause* of uterine (or any other) cancer, doctors believe it is safer to use oestrogen in a way that precludes any risk even of hyperplasia. To do this, administration of oestrogen must always be intermittent (usually three weeks on, one week off) so that in the week off medication the oestrogen level can decline as it regularly does in a woman's natural monthly ebb and flow of hormones. If there has been a build-up of uterine lining, then this pause usually allows it to regress, but as a further insurance some doctors also like to prescribe the second female sex hormone, progesterone, to be taken alongside oestrogen over the last five to seven days of the cycle. The presence of the progesterone simulates the natural hormone pattern at this stage of the monthly cycle, and cuts out all risk of hyperplasia by inducing shedding and light menstruation within one to three days of both oestrogen and progesterone tablets being stopped.

Providing oestrogens are administered on a cyclic basis, most gynaecologists today dismiss the cancer risk completely, and indeed the British Committee on the Safety of Medicines have issued a firm statement, exonerating both oestrogens and progesterone from any causal relationships with cancer.

Quite apart from the convincing figures showing the re- duced incidence of cancer in women on long-term oestrogen replacement, there is also more general evidence to be deduced from the fact that despite increased use of oestrogens over the last twenty years, uterine cancer figures are declining and breast cancer remains unaltered. It could be significant too that women tend to develop cancer when there is *less* oestrogen in their bodies, not when there is more. During pregnancy, when a woman's ovaries pour out enormous quantities of oestrogen (often six hundred times as much as normally) the incidence of breast cancer is actually less than with non- pregnant women, and this applies equally to women who have several children in rapid succession, thus keeping up an almost continuous high level of oestrogen. Conversely over 90% of cancer comes after forty, at a time when oestrogen levels are declining. Some doctors believe that the lowered oestrogen levels may be a factor in reducing the efficiency of the immune system, but the whole mechanism of ageing with faulty copying of cells is too complex (and still too little understood) for firm conclusions to be drawn.

The second objection doctors raise is one which Great Britain has always taken more seriously than any other country – that is, the increased thrombosis risk relating to oestrogen and the contraceptive pill. The World Health Organization actually estimates this to be five to eight times higher for women on the old high dosage pills than for the other women of similar age in the population.

Because the risk has been found to be dosage related, new low-dosage contraceptive pills have been developed. For replacement therapy at the menopause the dosage of oestrogen required is lower still, but even more important *natural* oestrogen can be used. This is not practical for oral contraception, as too much would be needed to prevent ovulation.

It was in Great Britain in 1968 that both the natural oestrogen (Premarin) and progestogen (synthetic progesterone) were exonerated of any effect on platelet behaviour. These 'platelets' are blood constituents, whose variable adhesiveness affects clotting potential, and the work showed that while synthetic oestrogens did adversely affect platelet behaviour making them 'stickier', natural oestrogen and progestogen did not. Although this work was published in *The Lancet* in June and August of 1968, few doctors appear to have read it or realized its importance.[7]

Since then more work has been done at the Addington Hospital, Durban, also checking the metabolic effects of Premarin, and this was reported at the 20th British Congress of Obstetrics. Again it confirmed no adverse effects either on platelets or any of the other coagulation factors tested.[8]

Similar work carried out in the UK with another naturally-occurring oestrogen, Harmogen (not yet published) has also revealed no significant changes in blood-clotting parameters, though in the same study the synthetic oestrogen, ethinyl-estradiol, was shown to produce slight changes in the direction of potential risk.

So once again this important difference between natural oestrogens and synthetic oestrogens was confirmed, and a leader in the *British Medical Journal* on the 9th February, 1974, further emphasized the point. Yet there are still doctors on both sides of the Atlantic who fail to recognize this, and the important safety factor involved.

It was important too that progestogen was also exonerated of affecting clotting potential, because as already mentioned many doctors favour the use of this alongside oestrogen at the end of each cycle to promote regular shedding of the endometrium.

This combined therapy not only cuts out the risk of hyperplasia, as we have seen, but by ensuring regular 'menstruation' during the week off all medication, it also eliminates the inconvenience of the occasional breakthrough bleeding, which can occur with a full replacement dosage of oestrogen on its own.

This tendency to breakthrough bleeding with prolonged use of oestrogens is the other argument which doctors use against the therapy. It does constitute a valid objection, because any unexpected bleeding demands investigation to eliminate any possible sinister cause.

Although the combined therapy successfully solves this problem from the doctor's point of view, not all women are prepared to accept even light and controlled bleeding. This is particularly true if there has been a long gap between finishing menstruation and starting HRT. Where the patient is adamant about this, she can be stabilized on a lower dosage of oestrogen which does not cause bleeding. Some doctors argue, however, that a very low dosage may not be fully effective in terms of the wide protection the therapy is designed to give.

The pros and cons of this, and women's own attitudes toward menstruation are discussed more fully later. For the moment in this chapter it is more important to analyse the attitudes of the doctors themselves, because even when they are satisfied about the cancer risk, the thrombosis risk and the management of bleeding, they still raise other objections.

Within any structure of socialized, free or insured medicine, one argument often heard is an economic one, with dire prophesies of the time and expense involved if any mass demand for HRT is encouraged.

While this may be particularly relevant under Britain's National Health Service, it does also affect attitudes in private medical insurance and within free clinics in the States. HRT can be obtained by non-paying patients at some of these clinics, but only where the doctor in charge is convinced of the urgent need for it.

One top London consultant explained his own different attitude toward free HRT for all menopause women. He admitted, 'The menopause is a hormonal deficiency, and if you accept this, then you accept it needs treatment like any other deficiency. There is overwhelming evidence of the benefits of such treatment, physically, psychologically and sexually, and there is no evidence at all of harmful effects.' But then he went on. 'It is one thing to prescribe this for patients paying for their own medication. It is another to envisage the Health Service coping with a large-scale mass demand, which would tax both our financial resources and our time. With both limited, one has to consider if a free contraceptive service, for example, should not take higher priority.'

The same sort of considerations must obviously affect private insurance schemes in the States. Certainly there appears to be considerable reluctance to include HRT in their benefits.

But the economic argument against HRT could be short-sighted. Doctors who do prescribe the treatment argue that it is actually far less costly than the Librium and Valium so freely dished out to menopausal women by other physicians, and they also argue that in the end it saves on doctor-hours by eliminating consultations in the short-term for the common menopause conditions such as flushes and depression, and in the long term for more serious problems.

In Japan one large industrial concern, at least, has come down in favour of HRT on economic grounds. At their own Medical Centre, HRT is given free to menopausal women employees as a means of cutting down on absenteeism.

But behind the medical and economic objections, sometimes lightly camouflaged by them and at other times quite openly trotted out as the clinching arguments, is the old 'interfering with nature' concept. Because sooner or later *all* women suffer from shrivelling ovaries and declining oestrogen, it is argued it must be natural and, therefore, right.

A logical extension of this argument would mean that other aspects of ageing which are universal, such as decaying teeth or failing sight, would also go untreated, or even that medical knowledge should not be used to combat the ultimate decline into death. Universality is a poor reason for non-treatment.

Women suffer very much from this attitude held by doctors. One wrote to me bitterly, 'The menopause has made my life a misery now for years. It has ruined for me and my husband what should have been our good years, with the children grown up and freedom to enjoy things before we are really old. Most of the time I feel too rotten and flushes and sweats sap my energy. All my doctor says is, "It is natural" and "It is just your age. I can't help you." Why should only menopausal symptoms be considered natural and go untreated?'

It is certainly arguable that if it were men who faced a physical menopause with atrophy of their sex organs in middle-age, the male-dominated medical profession would long since have done something about it. There would certainly be far less talk about it being natural and right.

So how natural is the menopause? What purpose does it serve? And why is the human female the only one in all nature to suffer the 'change of life'?

7. The menopause and evolution

In the whole of nature, only the human female suffers a physical menopause. While other animals remain potentially fertile until death, a woman is deliberately programmed for her ovaries to shut down in mid-life. When the number of eggs stored in the ovaries has declined to a certain level, new orders are triggered for the ovaries to cease to produce oestrogen. Finally they atrophy and shrivel, bringing an end to her fertile life.

The age at which this usually happens has always been between forty-five and fifty. Aristotle who lived over three hundred years before Christ wrote, '... for the most part fifty marks the limit of women's reproductive capacity.' Avicenna, a famous Arab physician of the eleventh century pointed out, 'There are women whose menstruation lapses quickly to end in their thirty-fifth or fortieth year, but there are others in whom it lasts until they reach fifty.'

There are many fantastic claims of late fertility, including the biblical story of Sarah bearing a child when over ninety. However, such reports from ancient times and civilizations where births and deaths were not officially registered as they are today are notoriously unreliable. The oldest, fully documented birth was to Mrs Ruth Alice Kistler of America, who is reported in the *Guinness Book of Records* as giving birth to a daughter on 18 October 1956, at the age of 57 years, 129 days.

At the other end of the scale, some women do suffer a very early menopause in the thirties, and occasionally ovarian failure may occur even before that.

Extensive records show that the age at which these fresh instructions begin to operate and the date of final menstruation, are closely linked in mothers and daughters, a fact which tends to confirm the genetic nature of the control underlying the process. Instances of premature menopause in the same family provide the most striking evidence of this. In one family three sisters are recorded ceasing menstruation at thirty-three, thirty-eight and thirty-three respectively, and their mother at forty-two.

It is interesting that modern records are now showing the average age for the menopause extended to over fifty-one, and with puberty also coming earlier, it would appear to indicate adaptation to the longer life-span by an extension also of female fertile life.

But why is the female blueprint designed in this particular way to set a limit on fertility? Why did evolution favour the female menopause in the human race? And why are women unique in this respect?

The reasons seem clear, if somewhat negative. The most important advantage was ensuring that ova which had been stored too long had no chance to be fertilized. There is a tendency for ova to deteriorate over the years and an example of this is the higher incidence of mongolism in babies born to older mothers, due to defective chromosomes in the female egg.

In contrast male sperm is not stored and is not, therefore, subject to the same risk of deterioration. It is freshly manufactured throughout life.

Another reason for limiting the period of fertility in women was to ensure that children should not be born to mothers unlikely to live long enough to rear them. The human child is dependent on its mother for many years, and in the past repeated and dangerous childbearing, lack of hygiene, poor nutrition and little medical knowledge meant that women died young. It seems incredible today to realize that at the time of the Roman Empire the average life expectancy for a woman was only twenty-five. By the time of the discovery of America it had increased to about thirty years, and even by the Victorian era it had only risen to forty-five.

Another and more subtle reason for the menopause put forward by one anthropologist was the need to ensure some older women surviving to pass on acquired female wisdom and skills. By eliminating the special hazards of late childbirth, there was an improved chance of a few old wise women living on to the benefit of both tribe and race. In such primitive times the only means of passing on knowledge was by example, demonstration or word of mouth. The 'elders' of a tribe had a special status and special services to render.

So in evolutionary terms it can be seen that the menopause had an important part to play. But it was important to the individual woman too. It brought the only relief then known from the tyranny of constant pregnancies. Some wit once declared that the safest form of contraception has always been the word 'No' spoken firmly, but in rougher and ruder times when women were merely possessions and wealth was counted in the number of sons, refusal had little effect on men who did not need to bother about the finer points of courtship or consent.

So, in the past, those women living beyond the menopause must have been mainly conscious of relief that the annual ordeal of childbirth appeared to be over.

The train of events that followed, the adverse effects on energy, health and appearance, were simply accepted as an inevitable part of ageing. Nature clearly lost interest in the infertile woman and saw no purpose in keeping her desirable, so the lack of oestrogen not only ended reproduction, but ended the positive effects on skin, muscle, and bone, allowing accelerated ageing to take place.

Alongside the compensation of being free of childbearing, a woman who survived beyond mid-life had to accept that she was old and had ceased to be sexually interesting. The menopause marked the end of her life as a desirable woman, and, since she could no longer produce sons, it also reduced her value as a wife.

One can imagine clear elements of personal tragedy in this for women, but for men it did not matter much. A man might get through several wives in the course of his life-time. His virility continued; he could go on enjoying sexual adventures and fathering children right into old age. He did not even have to bother about retaining youthful good looks and figure. This was not demanded as part of male attraction, as it was (and still is) demanded as part of female attraction. So the extraordinary double standards of behaviour and appearance, which we have come to take for granted, can be seen to be rooted to quite a large extent in the phenomena of the menopause, and in the striking contrast it produces in the way men and women age.

But because the majority of women did not survive long beyond the menopause anyway, and because it involved little or no inconvenience to the male, who had the money and power to decide the direction of any research, the menopause attracted little or no attention socially or medically until quite recently.

It is extraordinary looking through the literature on the subject to discover how little was really understood about the menopause and associated female phenomena until this century.

Because the menopause was seen as a negative thing, basically as the absence of the monthly 'issue of blood', folklore about it is inextricably linked with the mythology of menstruation, though assuming the opposite interpretations. So to understand attitudes to the menopause, it is necessary to understand attitudes to menstruation.

In the very beginning, because blood was associated in the primitive mind with wounds, injuries and death, menstruation was viewed with fear and superstition. It became the subject of strict taboos in every culture, and there is still an echo of this in our own rational age in the lingering use of the old euphemism, 'the curse'.

Pliny, who lived from AD 23 to 79, wrote many books, among them one called *Natural History*, which has been described as the first encylopaedia. In it he points out that menstruating women had disastrous effects on quite ordinary things. They not only turned wine sour and seeds sterile, but caused grass and garden plants to wither and fruit to fall from any tree beneath which they sat.

In ancient times menstruating women were so much objects of dread that in many cultures there was a prohibition against any contact with them, and in some parts of the world they were even segregated into special huts, built at some distance from the villages.

They were obliged to call attention to their condition by smearing bright coloured dyes on their faces or wearing masks, and even calling out 'Unclean, unclean'. In Mosaic law a woman had to be put apart for seven days at the time of menstruation, and anyone or anything she touched became equally contaminated.

It is no surprise to find Christianity inheriting these old

beliefs and forbidding women to enter sacred buildings while menstruating. But the superstition also extended into commerce, with menstruating women forbidden to work in sugar refineries in France, as they were thought to turn the sugar black. In Mexico the same ban applied to women working in the silver mines, as they caused the ore to disappear, while in Indo-China no woman was employed in the opium industry for fear that menstruation would turn the opium bitter.

To us now it seems just ancient rubbish but the idea persisted strongly for centuries, and as recently as 1878 a physician wrote to the *British Medical Journal*, reporting two instances where hams had been spoiled because a menstruating woman had cured them.

In the remoter parts of England and Wales, it is still possible to find women being advised during menstruation not to touch red meat for fear it should 'go off', not to attempt to make bread because the dough would not rise, and never, never, for some inexplicable reason, to touch salt.

To the ancients the actual cause of menstruation was a complete mystery and it was blamed variously on gods, evil spirits, crocodiles, birds and the moon. The fact that it occurred at roughly four-week intervals strongly favoured the moon theory, and Aristotle asserted the moon was female because 'the menstrual flux and the waning of the moon both take place towards the end of the month, and after the wane and discharge both become whole again'.

The patent absurdity of a theory which would make all women menstruate at the same time seems to have worried very few people, and the superstition constantly reappeared. In 1704, no less a person than Richard Mead, physician to the English King, George II, wrote, 'In countries nearest the Equator where we have proved lunar action to be strongest, these monthly secretions are in much greater quantity than in those near the poles where the force is weakest.' Even more unbelievably, as recently as 1938, American medical students could still read in one of their most authoritative textbooks of obstetrics that 'over 71% of women menstruate every twenty-eight days and the majority during the new moon'.

Although the moon was believed to have such influence in

triggering the event, the purpose was widely believed to be a form of purging, by which women were relieved of impurities and excess blood. The belief that the flow contained poisonous material underlies more superstitions, and there is even, strangely, some modern support for this concept of a toxic substance, with women reporting that flowers fade, particularly if worn in a corsage, during the menstrual period. The theory put forward is that this toxic substance at such times also invades the perspiration.

Getting nearer the truth, but still vague and inaccurate, were the ideas of Hippocrates, the father of medicine, who at least groped toward the relationship between menstruation and reproduction with his theory that the menstrual flow was the nourishment which fed the child. Pliny went further, believing it was the actual substance from which the child was shaped and formed.

Whatever the view favoured, the opposite of menstruation, the cessation of the menstrual flow was still a bad thing. It meant that woman was no longer getting rid of her 'evil humours' and the poisons were building up inside her, or it meant she no longer produced the substance of life. Either way she was diminished. She was no longer a real woman.

Margaret Mead, the famous American anthopologist, makes this point in her book *Male and Female*. She found that both pre-pubertal girls and post-menopausal women in many societies were treated as men. Referring to the social role of women after the menopause, she writes,

Where reproductivity has been regarded as somewhat impure and ceremonially disqualifying – as in Bali – the post-menopausal woman and the virgin girl work together at ceremonies from which women of child-bearing age are debarred. And she adds, Where modesty of speech and action is enjoined on women, such behaviour may no longer be asked from the older woman, who may use obscene language as freely as or more freely than any man.

This loss of femininity after the menopause and the change to neuter or masculine role is not only enshrined and emphasized by cultural attitudes and superstitions, but is something deeply felt by women, particularly the more uneducated and unsophisticated, whose role and status has been largely confined to the domestic and maternal. Such women vaguely envisage 'the change' as meaning real anatomical or structural changes taking place, and one seventy-year-old woman actually believed that women turned into men inside. She insisted she had been aware of this process taking place and had felt it as a 'turning and tightening of the thigh muscles'.

In his excellent booklet *The Menopause – a neglected crisis*, Robert G. Richardson writes,

We must ask why an event of such significance to the individual woman passed almost without notice sociologically, anthropologically and medically. And the answer thrown back from the silent past is that the menopause was a negative event of no importance in the life of the community. So when a woman's usefulness was seen to be ended, she ceased to be a woman.

In the under-populated ancient world a woman's usefulness was measured by her fertility. In our modern crowded world the time is fast approaching when infertility in itself becomes a virtue. Certainly the fifty-plus woman today is no longer on the discard heap. Her wisdom, skill, experience and energy are badly needed and she becomes relatively 'young' in a population living to a new time-scale, which means that in the USA alone there are twenty-two million people aged over sixty-five.

Of course, with their conscious and reasoning minds women realize how much things have changed. They recognize their own value today to their families and to society. But beneath the surface old atavistic memories linger and lurk. And, amazing, as it may seem, some women today still give credence to dark notions that the menopause can cause them to lose their minds. They fear emotional and mental instability. Such a belief could be rooted in the very real evidence of depression and confusion, which glandular imbalance can produce, but it almost certainly also stems from deeper hidden memories of a time when it was believed that the ageing female body could no longer expel the 'evil humours' in the cleansing monthly flux.

So science may banish superstition, modern medicine eliminate the menopause, but old attitudes persist. Too many women still today feel diminished and threatened by the change of life.

They fear not only mental and emotional instability, but actual sexual inadequacy, lack of response and loss of attraction.

It is fear of the castrating effect of the menopause plus the onset of emotional instability which, according to popular novels, drives previously respectable women to seek erotic adventures before the menopause robs them of all sexual satisfaction.

The middle-aged woman, hitherto of impeccable character, who goes off the rails, falling victim either to the attractions of a young lover or the blandishments of a suave adventurer is an accepted figure. But she is not really very true to life according to Dr Isabel Hutton. In her book *The Hygiene of the Change in Women* she writes,

Popular novels often give the impression that women are unduly amorous at this time and inclined to break loose from all decorum. We are familiar with the kind of literature in which women, at what is called 'the dangerous age' fall in love with young men and make themselves ridiculous with their overtures. These novels lead us to suppose that women are pursuing a last love affair before reaching the age which is supposed to be the end of their sex-life.

In all the writer's experience, not a single case of this kind, directly attributable to the climacteric has ever been met with. An amorous, flighty woman will continue so throughout the 'change of life' and afterwards, but she does not suddenly develop these characteristics between forty and fifty years of age.

Maybe the onset of the menopause does not change basic moral values, but it certainly can change a woman's nature in other ways. The letters I receive make it clear that many women at this time become irritable and difficult to live with. What is more, they are aware of this and worry about the effect on their family, but seem powerless to do anything about it. HRT helps by restoring hormonal balance, which in turn soothes the disturbed nervous system.

In his booklet on the menopause, Robert Richardson points out that not surprisingly, in view of their scientific interest during the nineteenth century, it was the French who incorporated these emotional aspects of the menopause into the literature of the period. He quotes from Octave Feuillet's comedy, *La Crise*, written in 1882. Julia, the heroine and a previously well-balanced personality, reflects:

C

What name can be given to this moral affliction, to this discontent with myself and with those about me that I have felt for some months. My husband is, doubtless, the best of men. But nothing that he says or does pleases me. His watch charms irritate me above all else. Yet these charms and I have lived together in peace for ten years. Then suddenly, one fine day, we hate each other. My husband has the insufferable habit of jingling them while he is talking – making an unbearable clinking. At the very instant that I write these lines he is in his room, winding his watch and making a noise with those charms.

Her husband, M. de Marsan, a magistrate, visits his doctor. It is not [he says] a question of extravagant symptoms that would attract the attention of outsiders, but of shades, each day more marked, which do not escape an intimate like myself. For ten years I have said I possessed a treasure in my life. Then suddenly this sweet Julia takes on the air of a martyr – obedient, but irritated. This woman of the world, this refined woman now speaks a language full of sharp, bitter words, harsh and peevish maxims. I find in her conversation – previously so mild – a banal melancholy, a sharp poetic flavour, with a socialistic tendency which fills me with uneasiness. . . . At the same time that the wife changed, the mother changed too. Her husband is now a tyrant, the children a heavy burden. She scarcely speaks to them. They are left to themselves. Here, then, doctor, is what happened to me. Here is the crown of thorns which Julia has put upon my innocent head, without the least provocation on my part. What is the explanation?

[The doctor replies]
Perhaps I have it – your wife's age . . . It is a normal disease that may attack the best of women as they reach threshold of maturity. Such is the attraction of the evil fruit which Eve held for the first time in her hands. Thus the most honoured woman may sense a desire not to be resigned to death without having tasted it.

Robert Richardson comments that thus, belatedly, both literature and medicine acknowledge that a woman's emotions are disturbed at the menopause and that, as Byron wrote in *Don Juan,* 'though her years were waning, her climacteric teased her like her teens'.

8. The menopause and the modern family

Today the fact that both her family and society accord the modern woman such an active and challenging role in middle-age, is far more a matter for congratulation than commiseration. To be thought young and to be encouraged to think of herself as young, is entirely on the credit side, but it does involve staying mentally and physically as fit as possible.

Very little attempt is made in the world today to cushion a woman through the menopause years or make life easier for her. Even if it were thought necessary, it would probably be difficult to achieve. The average family can neither afford nor obtain paid help, and the unpaid sort, once given by aunts, cousins and parents, usually living just around the corner, has vanished along with the extended family. Our industrialized and mobile society has brought not only dispersal of the family, but of the close-knit village community, once another source of support.

It has also brought a vast speeding up in communications, ideas and rates of change, so that the gap in thinking and attitudes between one generation and the next has widened to put the whole fabric of the family under stress. In the past, within the family and within society itself, roles and rules were sharply defined; parents were obeyed, elders respected and children protected. Each person knew his place, and few dared try to leave it or to question existing conditions and values. This whole safe, solid structure was firmly buttressed externally by the laws of church and state.

Today the middle-aged woman has no such certainties in her life and no simple rules either to live by herself, or to help her bring up her children. All authority is questioned and by the onset of the menopause, she can find herself firmly stuck in a peculiar 'middle-aged sandwich', caught between worries over her adolescent children on one side, and problems starting to arise with her ageing parents on the other.

In addition to her complex role in the home, if she also

does a full or part-time job, she may well be facing extra problems at work as she reaches positions of greater responsibility.

In 1890 in America only 6% of married women worked. Today fifteen million women of forty-five or older, most of them married, are employed full-time, and over 50% of married women do paid or voluntary work.

The percentage of married women doing jobs in Great Britain is much the same, and so are their reasons for working. Although only 44% are officially registered as paid workers, many more do small part-time jobs and voluntary welfare. Where once the reasons for working were almost always economic, women today work just as much for fulfilment, to use their education and training, or simply to help combat the new loneliness and loss of identity which seems so much part of urban living.

But the modern woman has yet another role, the sexual role. This again is in striking contrast to her mother and grandmothers, who in the middle-class society in Victorian times were thought far too spiritual and delicate actually to enjoy anything so coarse as sex. In an age when even piano legs were considered improper and had to be covered with frills, it was not surprising that a woman's body should be a secret and a slightly shameful mystery, while sex for a 'nice' woman was something to be endured rather than enjoyed. One British aristocrat was supposed to have observed that during sexual intercourse 'a true lady never moves'.

That story is probably apocryphal, but it does indicate the prevailing attitude. A lady was not expected to be skilled in sex, initiate it, enjoy it, or even be responsive. She was not an equal sexual partner. Today she is. She has been taught to accept and even take some pride in her own sexual nature, and positively conditioned to expect pleasure as well as to give it.

In her middle-years, relieved of the fear of pregnancy and the need to 'take precautions', women often experience a new surge of interest in sex. Above all they have a new need for it. With the children gone from home, they often suffer a sense of loss, of not being needed any more, and there can be compensation and comfort in being needed by their sexual partner.

At just the time when this sexual bond can be of special

help, unfortunately the menopause can produce both physical and psychological complications. Dr William H. Masters, Director of the Reproductive Biology Foundation in St Louis, Missouri and famous co-author with Virginia Johnson of *Human Sexual Response* and *Human Sexual Inadequacy*, believes that the psychological pressure of society's attitudes toward the menopause adversely affect women in their sexual response at this time.

He said,

Many women approach the menopausal years with grave concern because they've absorbed a lot of nonsense that goes along with our society's concept of the menopause. You're finished, you're through as a woman – that sort of thing. If women are concerned, if they are fearful, if they feel that they are less than complete individuals as they go through the menopause, then of course these concepts can affect sexual function. Anything that makes one question one's sexual effectiveness can interfere with responsivity.

The point at which sexual activity may decline depends on the information and attitudes of both husband and wife. Given a reasonably healthy male as an interesting and interested partner, there is no reason why effective sexual function can't continue for women into the seventy- and eighty-year-old group. Unfortunately it is widely believed that a post-menopausal woman loses her ability to respond sexually. Of course this is nothing more than a great cultural fallacy.

Some women certainly are reputed to retain sexual interest and drive late into life. Princess Metternich, when asked at what age a woman ceases to be capable of sexual love is supposed to have replied, 'I do not know, I am only sixty-five.' Simone de Beauvoir quotes an old lady of eighty, asked the same question, who also said, 'You will have to ask someone older than I.'

It would be interesting to know if there is any correlation between women who remain sexually active and possession of adrenal glands which maintain high oestrogen levels.

As we have seen, the opposite can be true. The shut-down of the ovaries and very low oestrogen levels can produce an atrophic state of the vagina which makes intercourse painful or sometimes impossible, with indirect reduction in libido.

Experts on sexual response such as Masters and Johnson were aware of this physical hazard of the menopause a quarter of a century ago, and were recommending oestrogen replacement therapy even then. Dr Masters said,

We use topical or systemic oestrogen replacement. Administration of adequate amounts of oestrogen reconstitute the pelvic tissues to a state akin to that of the pre-menopausal years. The vaginal mucosa thickens, the lubricative pattern develops with more facility and earlier in the response cycle. A great deal of vaginal distensibility is returned. The uterus returns to a pattern of regularly recurrent contractions rather than a spasm with orgasm, and there is a significant increase in blood supply to the pelvis, which facilitates the rapidity and degree of the female's response. We generally use the oral form of replacement with natural oestrogen and continue it indefinitely.

The story of Frankie Fullam and her husband illustrates graphically the sort of problems the menopause can bring into the life of an ordinary married couple. Frankie and Bill quite deliberately describe themselves as 'ordinary', middle-class and middle-income. Bill was a POW in Japanese hands during the war, but he made a good recovery and settled down to a modest job in the Civil Service. They had one son, now grown up. Perhaps the thing not quite so ordinary about them is their obvious and unembarrassed love for each other. Probably only the strength of this got them through the first terrible years of the menopause before Frankie found out about Hormone Replacement. She described to me exactly what happened.

My periods began to get less in 1965 when I was only forty-five and I began to get awful headaches for which my doctor gave me painkillers. By September 1966, my periods had stopped and I remember my first thought was how lovely to be able to have intercourse without precautions at last. But by Christmas my headaches were terrible and I began to have dizzy spells and blackouts. I went back to my GP in the New Year, and when I told him the periods had stopped he confirmed it was the 'change of life' and 'all quite natural'. He gave me stronger tablets but I felt no better, and had to give up my part-time job as I just couldn't concentrate. I was also getting palpitations which scared me.

The headaches were so severe that my own doctor finally sent me to hospital for tests and X-rays. Again I was told it was just 'the change' and nothing was wrong with me.

As the months went by I started hot flushes and awful vaginal irritation. I was given cream and painkillers but by now I was spending days in bed, feeling really ill, and my husband had to lose time off work to look after me. When I did get up, I would look at myself in the mirror and see an old woman, with dry grey-looking skin. It was not a bit like me, and I really felt like doing away with myself. If I had not had such a good husband, I would have done.

As the years went by I experienced night-sweats so severe I had to get up many times during the night and dry myself down. My husband and son by then had got used to getting their own breakfast and sandwiches. I just couldn't do it for them.

Then intercourse started to become painful and I found myself dreading my husband making love to me. The vagina was dry and unyielding and, sensing I could not respond, Bill didn't bother me. I lost all feeling in the breasts too, so that love-play had no meaning for me.

When my husband asked our GP if I was a sick woman, he said, 'Oh no, she is only going through the menopause. It is all quite natural. It is lucky she is not an invalid as many women are during the change.'

This went on for seven years until in 1973, Frankie read my series on Hormone Replacement in the *London Evening News*. She took the articles to her doctor, who told her firmly that it was nonsense, that she had enough oestrogen in her body, and hormone pills would only throw the balance out and give side-effects. He said 'the change' could go on for ten years and offered her more drugs.

But by now Frankie and Bill had had enough. They went to a doctor privately who specialized in HRT. Full tests were carried out and Frankie's oestrogen level was found to be more or less nil. He also confirmed that the vagina had shrunk and this was causing the pain during intercourse. He put Frankie on natural oestrogen and told her to come back in six weeks. She told me what happened next.

The only side-effect for me was slight indigestion in the first few days. Within the six weeks my headaches, flushes, night sweats and palpitations had all gone.

I saw the specialist again and he remarked how different I

looked. My skin was better, I was less tense, and he renewed the prescription for a further three months.

Well, within that time I was feeling sexy and wanting to go to bed with my husband again. You can imagine the joy for both of us after those dreadful years. My breasts had firmed up, the vagina was moist again and there was no discomfort at all when we made love.

Ever since we have had a wonderful life again. I feel young and attractive, my hair has thickened up and my skin is really good. I have masses of energy and it is wonderful to be so well after so long feeling only half a woman and half alive. I am doing a part-time job once more.

I have no side-effects and no withdrawal bleeding on my regime of one tablet a day for twenty-one days, then a week off. When I had a smear test after a year on this treatment, the young doctor would not believe I was nearly fifty-five. My oestrogen level was pre-menopausal. What staggers me is that my own GP, who admits that I look marvellous and that the treatment has done wonders for me, will still not use it for his other patients.

Bill Fullam gave me an interesting view of the husband's bewilderment and misery when severe menopausal problems beset a marriage.

It is terribly puzzling for a man and difficult to know what to do for the best. Frankie used to get in the most awful moods, and would shout at me for no reason at all. She knew she was behaving badly but couldn't stop herself.

I spent days at home because she was too ill to get out of bed and scared to be on her own. I tried humouring her and I tried being firm, telling her to get a grip on herself. To be fair, she tried, but the next bout of headaches and hot flushes would be even worse. I found making her suppress her feelings aggravated things, and decided her tantrums and tears were a safety-valve.

We kept thinking it would all be over soon and that life would become tranquil and just right between us again, but instead it got worse. She'd be drenched in sweat at night and the doctor just kept on giving her tranquillisers and painkillers. When the vaginal trouble started I more or less stopped trying to make love to her.

That was the position for seven years until she went on oestrogen therapy. Since she was put on oestrogen, she has become cheerful and full of energy, and our love-life is better than it has ever been. But she is also serene and happy and there are no more arguments. In fact Frankie now is the woman I first married.

Frankie had a comparatively early menopause starting at forty-five, but for some women it can come even earlier, either naturally or as a result of surgical removal of the ovaries.

Joan Coady, an attractive and vivacious American woman living just outside New York told me she began 'the change' when only twenty-eight. She explained,

I became very depressed and my menstrual cycle was irregular. I put on weight, couldn't sleep and didn't want to meet people, to the point of becoming a recluse.
None of this was a bit like me and I lost all interest in sex, which wasn't like me either. I dragged from doctor to doctor, without getting any real help, then I happened to read Dr Wilson's book *Feminine For Ever*, and realised it could be a very early menopause. I went to a doctor who specialised in oestrogen therapy, and he confirmed I had an ovarian deficiency which had caused my low oestrogen level and early change of life. He prescribed natural oestrogen and I've never looked back. I am thirty-seven now and my children fourteen and fifteen. There just aren't enough hours in the day for all I want to do. The whole family has reaped the benefit of this therapy and of my feeling so well again. Certainly our sex life is better than ever.

The complete change in personality and the effect of this on the family was emphasized in another letter from a woman who had had her ovaries removed. She wrote,

I changed completely after the operation. I am not the same person. I used to be fun to live with, now I know I must be hell. I feel I have driven my children away from home and I can't blame them. When I complained to my doctor, he simply said, 'After what you had done, you can't expect to be the same.'

An early natural or surgical menopause is a very strong and direct indication for HRT. As one British gynaecologist put it, 'The earlier the menopause, the more prolonged and acute the changes and this can put a great strain upon a marriage if replacement therapy is not given.'

So many letters make clear how concerned women are for their families. A British woman wrote,

I am forty-seven and just starting the menopause. I am finding life grim with migraine, palpitations and night sweats. My doctor only gives me painkillers, and the depression and apathy I feel are affecting both my marriage and my job. My poor husband has reached the stage when he waits for me to speak first in case he upsets me in some way. I get very aggressive towards him. My job, which carries a great deal of responsibility, is also suffering. I have difficulty in applying my mind and making decisions.

Another British woman wrote,

Since my ovaries were destroyed by radium some six years ago, I have fluctuated in moods right down to absolute depression. This coupled with migraine, and arthritis in hips and knees (none of which I had ever experienced before) have all combined to reduce me from a basically light-hearted extrovert to a near-neurotic. The thing that worries me most is the effect on the family. It is changing the whole atmosphere of our home. I did suggest to my GP that hormone deficiency might be a contributory factor, but was told he wouldn't give me anything that might 'hold up the change'.

Both these women were intelligent and determined, but neither of them could persuade their own doctor to put them on HRT. In the end both had to change to doctors who prescribed Hormone Replacement Therapy, which in both cases proved a complete answer.

Time and again women have emphasized the effect of their own menopause problems on their adolescent children, with minor mutinies blown up into something far more serious by their mishandling or over-dramatizing of the situation. One mother wrote,

I can see now that it was my irrational behaviour which finally drove our daughter away from home. My mixture of tears and tantrums made her life a misery. Now after only a few months on oestrogen I am my old self again with the hot flushes, depression and exhaustion all gone, but the damage is done. If only I had known about HRT before so that the unnecessary rows and pre-mature break-up of the family could have been avoided.

One concerned daughter actually wrote to me herself putting the family problem. She stated,

My mother is forty-seven and has had all the menopause symptoms described for the last two years. She is very 'touchy' and yet the next minute can be in floods of tears. When she consulted her doctor she was fobbed off with 'It is your age', which was not a very comforting attitude. Could you let us have the address of a clinic?

Often it is clear that jobs as well as family suffer. Women in the teaching profession, particularly those in mixed schools, find menopausal flushes embarrassing and menopausal confusion and lack of confidence very detrimental to their work. But it applies in ordinary business life too. One woman wrote,

I have recently turned down a good post because I know that when I flush from the toes upwards, and feel like crawling into a corner, I just could not face a large office. So although I have the ability and could earn a great deal more, I stay in my safe little job and resign myself to that.

Another woman who had always helped her husband in the family business wrote,

Each visit my doctor told me my symptoms were natural at my age. I was then forty-three and he advised me to make one room in my house my private retreat and to spend most of my time there away from the demands of the family. As I help my husband run our business, I didn't seem able to impress on him that I just wanted the strength to live normally. All he gave me was Valium to help me sleep and some tablets for energy which sent me so demented that my husband stopped me taking them. I could no longer drive a car, which had been necessary in our business, and my days were a succession of incompleted tasks. Forgetfulness was now added to the nightmare and I wondered if it was premature senile decay.

After she had been put in touch with a clinic this same woman wrote again,

Only to let you know I have been on HRT for almost two cycles. The change is miraculous both physically and mentally. I can now do a really good day's work. I can plan my life and cope with my problems and feel better than I have felt for years.

So HRT is clearly the answer in many cases where the menopause appears to threaten a woman, her family or her job. But in Great Britain at the moment there is the question of availability, and this problem will be discussed in greater detail in the final chapter. Certainly at the moment a woman may have to be both determined and enterprising to obtain it, if her own doctor is uncooperative.

American women are amazed to hear of the problems British women face in getting oestrogen therapy. As one of them explained,

I simply told my doctor, when I knew the menopause was starting, that I wanted to be put on replacement hormones. He was not too keen at first, but I simply told him if he didn't give it me, I should go elsewhere. I knew a lot of my friends were on it and got it from their doctors. Now my own doctor has become convinced about the benefits, seeing how well it works for me and he prescribes it for other patients.

This sort of successful pressure on the doctor to comply with a patient's wishes is very alien to British medicine and certainly could not operate under the National Health Service. While middle-income American women automatically go to a gynaecologist for all their female problems, the British woman and her family is usually registered under the HNS with a local General Practitioner and only sees a specialist on his recommendation, if something arises which requires special investigation, treatment or surgery.

The final chapter will offer a more detailed comparison of the systems, but apart from any financial advantage to the patient in the British system, there is the advantage of the GP knowing the whole family and the circumstances in which they live, which can be relevant to appropriate medical treatment and decisions.

But the disadvantage is that the GP can too often be a complete autocrat. He does not *have* to consider his patient's wishes, and with only a small per capita payment under the NHS for each patient registered with him, regardless of the number of consultations, he may be only too willing to let an awkward or demanding menopausal patient go elsewhere quite unregretted. He will certainly not change his views or go even half-way to meet her wishes. If this is because they conflict with his deeply-held informed professional opinion, he is obviously justified. If they merely conflict with vague uninformed prejudice, he is not.

While the American woman can often pressure her doctor into trying her on HRT, pressure under the British system of socialized medicine seems to work very much the other way, with the patient hesitating to offend the doctor who looks after her whole family, and afraid in crowded urban areas of trying to change doctors because of the very real difficulty of finding another one to take them on.

It is a measure of the depth of desperation and strength of feeling among women on this issue of Hormone Replacement at the menopause, that so many of them do change their doctors as the only way of getting the treatment. It is also a measure of the change education has brought about in the attitudes and status of women that so many are no longer prepared to be treated, as one woman put it, 'as mindless idiots who have no right to be told anything and who must simply obey their doctors without explanation or question'. Another put it even more succinctly, 'Some doctors seem to feel a woman should only open her mouth to swallow his pills.'

9. Oestrogens, ageing and depression

It would be a pity if the criticisms made in this book of some doctors' attitudes toward their patients and toward their menopause problems, should suggest any bias on my part against the profession in general. On the contrary, in the years researching and writing on medical and social problems, I have found doctors to be almost without exception, truly concerned for their patients, dedicated to their work, and remarkably long-suffering with a lay journalist seeking knowledge. They are also blessed, and no doubt need to be, with a special and delightful sense of humour, which helps to lighten what must at times be a grim occupation.

One example of this was the wry joke told me by Sir John Peel, the Queen's former gynaecologist, now retired. We were discussing the need for women to come to terms with ageing, when he suddenly popped in the not entirely relevant story of the man who had suffered his first heart attack and asked his doctor what he should do about sex. 'No excitement, old man,' the doctor replied, 'stick to the wife.'

I appreciated that story. I also appreciated Sir John Peel's fair and sane approach to Hormone Replacement Therapy. Here was a man at the very top of his profession, a truly establishment figure, who was still prepared to allow me to quote him on this controversial question. He told me,

I have used natural oestrogen and cyclic combined hormone therapy for patients over quite long periods, for as much as ten years in some cases. There is no doubt it is of immense clinical benefit to some women between the ages of forty-five and fifty-five and does slow down some ageing processes for a time. Generally my patients are prepared to call a halt themselves at around sixty and I prefer this. At that point they are perhaps more ready to accept ageing.

Sir John's reservations about continuing the therapy into old age are rooted in the fact that other ageing processes still go on, and he, therefore, questions the value of the American rationale of 'oestrogen for ever'. He also insists that the really long-term effects of HRT continued into old age are not yet known.

In America in particular, I did meet many women who had been on oestrogen replacement for over twenty years and were still thriving on it well into their seventies and eighties. One of them was Robert Wilson's own wife, Thelma. It is always a good test of a doctor's faith in his own treatment if he uses it on his own family, and this pioneer of HRT was certainly not afraid to prescribe the treatment for his own wife in the very early days when it was still highly controversial medicine. After over twenty years on cyclic HRT, and now seventy-two Thelma Wilson remains healthy, active and looking far younger than her years. She still travels widely, researching and lecturing for the Wilson Foundation, and enjoys walking, golf and painting in her spare time.

Equally striking was Dr Jessica Marmoston, aged seventy-one, whom I met at the University of Southern California County Medical Center. The normal retiring age is sixty-five, but Dr Marmoston still retains her position as Senior Attendant Physician and Clinical Professor of Medicine. She lives in Los Angeles with her famous film-producer husband, Lawrence Weingarten, and takes a swim in her pool most mornings before setting out for the ten-mile drive to the hospital. She told me,

I have used oestrogen myself since I was forty-five. I have three children, now grown up of course, but I have always led a very busy life. Oestrogen therapy not only eliminates the usual meno-pausal symptoms, as I've proved personally and in my clinics, but researches in my own Heart Clinic have shown that oestrogens reduce the risk of arteriosclerosis and heart trouble. Oestrogen therapy seems to have some influence on the incidence of cancer in post-menopausal women. Of four hundred such women under treatment in our clinic, one half were given oestrogens and the other half were not. Only one incidence of cancer occurred among the oestrogen-treated patients, and that had occurred prior to therapy in an organ which does not respond directly to oestrogen. In contrast, seven cancers occurred in the patients not receiving oestrogen and two died. I still use oestrogen and it continues to give me the energy to cope with long hours. Often when I get home from the hospital there is still a great deal of work to be done in preparation for next day's clinic.[1]

Of course get-up-and-go is very much an American characteristic anyway, but it seemed particularly abundant in women
on HRT, even in the older groups.

But in England too, I met a remarkable seventy-three-year-
old doctor, who looked twenty years younger than her age,
and who had been on oestrogen for well over twenty years.
Dr Greta Malmberg told me,

I started with small doses of synthetic oestrogens to reduce menopausal problems, but later I read in a public health journal about
a doctor in the London area, who was using natural oestrogen on a
cyclic basis and I could see the medical logic of this concept. I
had married late to a man nine years younger than myself, so that
I had specially good reasons for wanting to keep young. . . .
I have been on a forty-two-day cycle for many years now and
feel absolutely fine. I work in school clinics and the Health Committee
retired me once because of my age, but I was clearly so fit that they
brought me back and I lead a busy professional life still, as well as
running my home.

The many women of this age on HRT, who keep fit, active
and interested in life, confirm the more scientific evidence of
the double-blind trials at Geriatric Centres, which established
the benefits of replacement therapy carried right on into old age.

Age is not a simple matter of years. It is a subtle interaction
between our physical and mental states and the amount of
involvement, interest and activity we are able to maintain.
American comedian, Jack Benny, was quoted as saying, 'Age is
a question of mind over matter. If you don't mind, it doesn't
matter', and there is a good deal of truth behind the quip.

It is much easier not to mind the facts of ageing if you feel
well enough and energetic enough to continue your interests,
maintain independence, retain identity and preserve dignity.

But with or without oestrogen therapy, in the present state of
medical knowledge, sooner or later the physical signs of ageing
have to be faced.

To the extent that HRT induces a sense of well-being and
renewed energy, to the extent that it keeps the vagina young
and healthy enabling normal sex life to continue, to the extent
that it keeps skin, hair and bone healthy, preserves muscle tone
and helps to check middle-aged spread, to this extent the
therapy can help to keep a woman young.

Obviously any cosmetic and rejuvenation effects of HRT are of immense importance to women, but advocates are usually careful not to over-stress them or suggest that oestrogen is some magic elixir of youth.

What oestrogen replacement can do is help a woman to age physiologically instead of pathologically. Robert Wilson himself put it to me in this way. He said,

We do not claim that cyclic oestrogen therapy rejuvenates or even prevents ageing, but it does slow it down, makes it a more gentle and gracious process, so that the way a woman ages parallels that of a man. There is no abrupt crisis, no total loss of femininity. Without this help, although modern diets, cosmetics and fashions may make a woman outwardly look even younger than her husband, her body still betrays her. She loses her confidence in herself at the very moment when she is free and most able to enjoy her life.

One of the ways in which accelerated ageing after the menopause makes a woman's body betray her, is in the effect of oestrogen deficiency on the skin, which becomes dry, papery and wrinkled. It can be a traumatic experience for a woman to look in her mirror in the cold light of day and see these changes. Vast sums of money are spent by women on various cosmetic techniques designed to conceal or rejuvenate. But the result, as one writer put it, is usually three stages of woman – childhood, youth, and 'you look wonderful'.

'You look wonderful' in this context too often only means 'You look wonderful for your age and full marks for trying'. But the woman in her fifties who has the time, money and motivation to take care of skin and hair can still only do so much. No amount of massage and make-up, however skilled, can fully camouflage the atrophic changes which take place in the tissues with age. Quite apart from the face itself, they show up relentlessly also on the skin of the neck, the inner arm and the inside of the thigh.

Hormone Replacement Therapy does seem to slow down these changes and the fact that oestrogen encourages a certain amount of sodium and water retention helps to prevent some wrinkling.

These cosmetic effects of HRT vary considerably from woman to woman, but in some they are dramatic. Although

Frankie Fullam was involved with the more serious problems of oestrogen deficiency, she found that oestrogen replacement not only solved these but also gave her the added bonus of improving skin and hair and generally making her look younger.

Another woman who described the cosmetic effects to me in detail was Mrs Elizabeth Vann, a fifty-two-year-old British housewife who had been on the therapy nearly three years. She also had a responsible job in the Civil Service and after she ceased to menstruate she ran into the common syndrome of depression, irritability and lack of confidence, all of which affected not only her home life but her job. She also told me she had begun to put on weight round the hips and thighs, her breasts had shrunk and her hair was lifeless and thinning.

Mrs Vann was put on a twenty-eight-day cycle of natural oestrogen, with a progestagen as well over the last five days. She told me,

My figure slimmed off again and my breasts improved. It sounds rather immodest but really HRT has done wonders for me. My hair is thick and glossy again and my skin marvellous. In particular that crêpey chicken look I was getting round the neck has disappeared. My legs which were flabby have firmed up and my hands, which have never been very good, have at least lost the wrinkly, veiny look. When I was out with my sister recently, who is six years younger than I am, I was taken for her daughter.

Although there is plenty of this sort of testimony and doctors too have noted from observation of patients that HRT usually improves elasticity and tone of the skin, there has not until recently been any actual scientific study. But at the International Health Foundation Workshop held in Geneva in 1972, Finnish gynaecologists, Professors Rauramo and Punnonen, reported experiments with three separate groups of fifty women, all of whom had had ovaries removed. In each case before the operation a piece of skin was taken from the thigh for biopsy, and thickness and rate of mitosis (cell division) measured.

A month after the operation, two of the groups were put each on a different oestrogen, while the third group went untreated.

At three months and again at six months, more skin was removed from a place adjacent to the first piece and further biopsy done. In the untreated women there was significant thinning of the epidermis and decrease in the rate of mitosis. In both groups of treated women there was actual thickening of the epidermis, no decrease in mitosis and clear indications that tissue changes were being prevented.[2]

The other way in which the body betrays the post-menopausal women, affecting health as well as mere vanity, is in weight increase and distribution. This was mentioned by Mrs Vann and was also one of the reasons why Betty Hilton Smart went on to HRT. As Betty Hilton, she was the leading British tennis player after the war, and still remains slim, athletic and attractive. She told me,

With the onset of the menopause for the first time in my life I felt tired and lacking in energy; I also found I was putting on weight. The whole medical concept of HRT seemed so logical to me that I got my doctor to refer me to a gynaecologist. Now I not only feel wonderful on oestrogen treatment, but my figure has firmed up again, and I am keeping my weight down to normal.

Body weight on average in women increases 12% between the age of twenty and sixty-five, then generally maintains a fairly constant level until the age of eighty when it begins to decrease again.

As with so many symptoms during the menopause, it is difficult to know just how much 'middle-aged spread' is due directly to changing habits and related ageing processes.

Older women do tend to take less exercise and are less active, which means less food is burned up as energy though they usually continue to eat just as much. In fact in some cases the joys of eating seem to become a form of compensation for other things they feel they are missing, and so food intake actually increases. This happens particularly with women who are bored and lonely, or who have perhaps become tired and discouraged by the obvious signs of ageing they perceive in themselves. One way and another it can add up to lack of motivation to restrict their diet or try to preserve their figure.

So far as I have been able to find out, only one controlled study has been done on weight increase in relation to HRT.

Dr Lauritzen, a gynaecologist attached to the University of Ulm, described at the Geneva Workshop how he had taken a group of 136 patients treated with natural oestrogen over a period of three years, and compared their weight increase in that time against a control group of untreated patients of the same age. He found that weight increases were significantly greater in the non-treated group.[2]

One bit of contributory evidence worth reporting, because it is so directly linked with oestrogens and ageing, is contained in experiments done at the University of Tokyo. Working there with female rats, Dr Hajimo Orimo showed that premature ageing, and in particular the increase of calcium deposits in tissues and organs, can be checked by administration of oestrogen.

It was already known that rats treated with the chemical, Dihydrotachysterol (DHT) for prolonged periods exhibited changes characteristic of premature ageing and very similar to the premature senility disease in humans, known as pregeria. These changes included atrophy and wrinkling of the skin, and arteriosclerosis with intense calcification of the arteries associated with shortened life-span.

Dr Orimo's deliberately 'aged' rats also showed atrophy of liver, kidney, skeletal muscle and adipose tissue, such as normally aged rats display, together with decrease in bone density and calcium content, suggesting osteoporosis. When natural oestrogen, Premarin, was administered alongside the DHT, the symptoms of premature old age did not appear. Dr Orimo concluded that his findings must encourage further study on the possibility of inhibiting the ageing process by administration of oestrogens.[4]

Again it is a big jump from rats to humans, but more and more ageing is being seen as a process probably originating at the cellular level which could have universal application. Women, unfortunately for their own peace of mind, are very different from rats and all other animals, in being conscious of their own ageing. In fact these changes in appearance, often coming quite suddenly after the menopause, can cause considerable distress, particularly in our present youth-orientated society.

Deterioration in hair, nails, skin and figure, however, even if accepted by doctors as related to oestrogen deficiency, are unlikely to be considered medically important, at least compared to serious effects of the menopause such as osteoporosis. And there is a curiously puritanical school of thought in medicine which questions the ethics of prescribing HRT simply to increase energy and well-being or to slow down ageing. These physicians question the right of any woman to receive treatment, unless she also displays severe classic menopause symptoms, such as hot flushes or vaginal atrophy.

Such attitudes are not only held by some elderly family doctors, who can be better forgiven for an old-fashioned medical and social stance, but with far less excuse by younger gynaecologists. Some women who have come up against this sort of attitude feel that occasionally it is rooted, albeit subconsciously, in male determination to keep the one biological advantage they have always had – their ability to age more slowly and retain sexual vigour longer.

Within the British National Health Service, where finance and facilities are limited and priorities compete and clash, a strong argument obviously exists for free HRT to be reserved for those who need it most and are suffering most.

But on a private and paying basis, if a woman wants HRT largely, or even only, because she feels it may help her to stay younger longer, then she surely has the right to buy it. If she is prepared to pay for the consultations, tests and yearly or twice-yearly follow-up, as well as her regular supply of oestrogen, this is her choice. And it is by no means the choice and perogative only of rich women, for in relative terms HRT is not an expensive procedure. It is comparable to the cost of the contraceptive pill, and a woman may well prefer to spend 25p a week on a supply of oestrogen rather than on cigarettes. There is no doubt which will do her more good.

In this connection there was a certain irony in my conversation with one young doctor. I had been invited to talk to a British Medical society, about Hormone Replacement Therapy. As we stood around afterwards discussing the pros and cons, one GP insisted strongly, 'I feel I should only prescribe oestrogen when it is absolutely necessary, and then for as short a time as possible. After all the long-term effects are still not really known.' As he spoke he was puffing away at a cigarette, apparently unconcerned about the *known* long-term effects of this drug on himself, or about the fact that he was forcing others to share the proven risk of lung cancer by polluting the air we all breathed.

Disentangling symptoms directly due to the menopause, from problems arising out of ageing and out of the normal stresses of life in the mid-years is always difficult. The truth is that both persist alongside each other in a sort of mutual aggravation. The already stressed situation makes menopausal problems worse, and the menopausal symptoms superimposed on the others often add up to a situation in which a woman carries a double load of depression, irritability, fatigue and insomnia.

Work done by Dr Jaszmann, a gynaecologist from Holland, was particularly revealing about these psychosomatic symptoms, previously dismissed by many doctors as not properly belonging to the menopause at all. Dr Jaszmann had the co-operation of some six thousand women all from one urbanized rural community and all between forty and sixty years. He divided them into biological age groups, according to how long it was since their last menstrual period. Then with their help he analysed and plotted as graphs the percentage of the women in each biological age group suffering from each symptom. The result was a series of lines peaking at certain times following final menstruation. For example hot flushes, pains in muscles and joints, formication and night sweats were all most frequently reported by women in the early post-menopause, and so the line for each of these symptoms peaked at a point within three years of ceasing to menstruate.

The psychosomatic symptoms, fatigue, headaches, irritability, dizziness and depression peaked much earlier when menstruation was starting to become irregular. Breathlessness, palpitations and actual mental unbalance did not show a real peak at all in any biological age group, and from this Dr Jaszmann concluded these symptoms were not truly menopausal. Sleeplessness showed a special pattern peaking five years after final menstruation but continuing high, so that it seemed to be a geriatric complaint rather than a solely post-menopausal one.[5]

The first real scientific evidence that depression can on occasions be linked with oestrogen deficiency came out of a series of double-blind trials carried out at the Merthyr Tydfil General Hospital, Glamorgan.

The Hamilton Depression Scale was used to score the severity of symptoms, oestrogen levels were established by vaginal cytology, and blood tests were also done to establish the level of free tryptophan (an amino-acid) in the blood. This bio-chemical aspect of the experiment was important, because previous work done by Dr Aylward and his team had shown that concentrations of free tryptophan in the blood were significantly lower in menopausal depressive patients than in corresponding controls. It had also established that certain natural oestrogens could increase the level of free tryptophan.

So a group of women were chosen who had had ovaries removed and who showed depression in addition to the usual accepted features of oestrogen deficiency. Initial blood tests established that the levels of free plasma tryptophan were significantly lower in this study group, than in a control group of women of similar age-range and socio-economic status, who were not depressive.

But after treatment for three months with an oestrogen (Harmogen) amounts of free plasma tryptophan in the study group were found to have increased to a point at which there was no significant difference in levels between them and the control group. What is more these same patients showed an improvement in depression, with scores which correlated with the increase in free tryptophan.

This research was particularly important not only because it showed that depression can be directly linked to lack of oestro-gen, but because it also indicated how the oestrogen-depression link may work through the influence of oestrogen in raising free plasma tryptophan levels. Finally, of course, it showed the administered oestrogen can also raise the tryptophan level and improve the depression.[6]

It is accepted, of course, that depression is more common following a surgical menopause than a normal one, and an interesting study confirming this was reported in *The Lancet* in August, 1973. Dr D. H. Richards gave the results of a follow-up on two hundred patients from his mostly urban group practice near Oxford, all of whom had had hysterectomies. Some sixty-five women had also had both ovaries removed and twelve others had had one ovary removed.

The two hundred patients were matched for age and as closely as possible for marital status etc., against two hundred female control patients, who had *not* had the operation.

Depression was defined for the purpose of the study as a condition which when diagnosed by any of the four partners in the practice, was treated with antidepressive drugs.

For 151 women, three years or more had elapsed since their operations, and fifty of them (33%) had depression within the three years, compared to only eleven (7%) of the matched controls. What is more nine of the hysterectomy patients required admission to mental hospital, as compared to only one of the controls.

The study showed depression after hysterectomy not only to be four times more frequent, but also more severe and of longer duration, lasting on average 24·6 months as against only 10·9 months in the control group. Almost half of the women developing depression after the operation did so within six months.

Dr Richard's own comments are interesting. He wrote,

The effect of hysterectomy seems in some respects to resemble that of the menopause, but in an exaggerated form. This view is further supported by the study of other signs and symptoms that are characteristic of women who have undergone hysterectomy. It is not uncommon for women who have had hysterectomy to suffer from hot flushes which begin shortly after their operation, irrespective of whether the ovaries have or have not been removed.

This and other symptoms raise the possibility that an endocrine factor may be involved even when the uterus alone is removed. Prospective studies are in progress to establish the degree and nature of endocrine change.

It would appear from this that removal of the target organ, the uterus, may in some way not yet understood, discourage the ovaries so that output is reduced and oestrogen levels drop. Or more prosaically, the surgery itself may simply have reduced blood supply to the ovaries, lowering their efficiency.

Whatever the reason may prove to be, if and when a hysterectomy does result in sluggish ovarian function, then obviously HRT is indicated. It is even more firmly indicated, of course, where the hysterectomy is accompanied by removal of both ovaries, producing a surgical menopause that often involves severe oestrogen deficiency symptoms.

Better understanding and greater usage of Hormone Replacement, together with refinements in methods of assessing hormone levels, both contribute today to more and more use of hormonal management to actually avoid the need for some hysterectomies.

Obviously where the symptoms, such as excessive bleeding or discharge are due to uterine disease, or where there are large fibroids, there is no alternative to surgery. In other cases where the underlying cause is faulty hormonal balance, then attempts should be made to correct this before the easier resort to the knife. There is some evidence that knife-happy surgeons too often remove symptoms by removing the uterus, without properly establishing the cause and considering alternatives. Critics insist that this is not only an easy way of avoiding time and trouble, but also an easy way of making money. But the opposing argument insists that the uterus serves no purpose other than to carry a baby for nine months, so that once the family is complete, if it is giving trouble it may as well be removed not only to overcome the present problems but to prevent future ones.

It is an appealing argument for the doctor, not quite so appealing for the woman who has to face the discomfort of the surgery and who rightly or wrongly resents losing an important part of her body that carried and nourished her children.

The answer has to be one based on medical knowledge and medical judgement, not on the patient's emotional reaction, but she is entitled to be sure that both judgement and knowledge are used on her behalf. Now it has been established that even simple hysterectomies can have a kick-back effect on the efficient working of the ovaries, there is even more reason for the pros and cons to be properly weighed up.

A letter stressing the effects of the loss of ovaries was sent to me by Joan Bates, a vicar's wife, living in Somerset. She wrote,

At the age of twenty-nine after only four years of marriage, I had to have both ovaries removed. We were very naive and went ahead at once to adopt a child. But after only six months I collapsed into severe depression. I loved my husband dearly, but experienced such a personality change that I told him to go away. I did not want to be his wife and I lost interest in him, my home, and life itself.

My local GP called in a psychiatrist and I was six months in a Psychiatric Unit, until in despair I left, with my husband being told there was 'nothing they could do'.

My husband refused to give up and quite by chance a friend told him of an endocrinologist. At St Thomas's Hospital in London I was put on hormone replacement with artificially induced menstruation. It has been miraculous and given us back a normal and happy married life. Over the years we have adopted three children, but I am convinced I could still be in a psychiatric hospital and on tranquillisers if it had not been for having a husband prepared to fight to get me HRT. I am sure there are many women in such hospitals today, being given the wrong treatment, when their depression like mine may be hormone-based.

Why are GP's so ignorant about it? American wives of Air Force men in this country have told me they cannot understand why so few English women know anything about oestrogen tests. They get their oestrogen levels checked regularly at the doctor's office on the Air Force Base. Here, doctors do not seem to recognise menopause symptoms half the time.

It is largely because the symptoms of the menopause appear at different biological ages, as Dr Jaszmann's work so clearly showed, that medicine has often failed to recognize them for what they are.

To some extent all tissues in the human body can be regarded as target organs for oestrogens, and the whole organism, therefore, reacts to oestrogen deficiency in varying degrees and at varying times. The hypothalmic centres are affected quickly so that hot flushes come early in the pattern, whereas bone tissues take a long time to be affected and so osteoporosis develops late.

This time-lag in the emergence of these symptoms, and the mixture of physical and psychic complaints, have confused diagnosis and blurred the picture so that doctors have recognized only part of it. In particular they have relied on tranquillizers to curb nervous effects, instead of oestrogens to eradicate them.

There has emerged a sort of half-way house in HRT, particularly perhaps in Great Britain, which has grudgingly accepted the value of oestrogen replacement in small doses and for short periods, and only to combat clear physical symptoms such as hot flushes and sweats. If as a by-product some of the psychosomatic symptoms are also relieved, there is a tendency to take this as proof that they were 'all in the mind', rather than accepting that these too had a hormone trigger.

What this form of short-term therapy does not take into account is that when it is stopped, the uncomfortable symptoms usually return, and even if they don't, other slow hidden degenerative processes associated with oestrogen deficiency go on.

So let us look at the ways in which Hormone Replacement Therapy is more properly used, and at the practical details of the tests, treatment and choices that face a woman and her doctor.

10. The test and the treatment

A changing menstrual pattern is usually a pretty firm indication that oestrogen levels are dropping. For many doctors this signal alone, or taken in conjunction with other menopause symptoms, is enough to allow replacement therapy to be started.

But other doctors like to employ a simple test actually to establish oestrogen levels. This not only provides a diagnostic confirmation but gives some indication of the oestrogen replacement dosage needed. Later on, when the test is repeated, it also serves to confirm that the replacement therapy is working satisfactorily.

The principle is simple. One of the main functions of oestrogen is to mature the cells of the vagina and keep it healthy and supple. A vaginal smear viewed under the microscope quickly reveals to the practised eye the number of mature cells, compared to the number of intermediate cells and immature cells. This ratio forms what is called the Maturation Index.

Hundreds of tests have already established that the Maturation Index for a normal, healthy, menstruating woman is in the area of eighty-five mature cells to fifteen intermediate with no immature cells. This figure varies slightly from woman to woman, and for some it may be nearer seventy-five mature to twenty-five intermediate, but there should be few or no immature cells so long as oestrogen levels are reasonably high.

For the untreated post-menopausal woman, however, the index can be completely reversed, so that there are few or no mature cells and the majority are intermediate or immature. A short time on oestrogen replacement usually brings the index back within the normal range, and this is a strong indication that the therapy is working correctly.

It is important, however, to emphasize that vaginal smears do not always correlate completely with menopause symptoms or with the patient's response to hormone therapy. This is because the smear can be influenced by many other factors, such as *when* it was taken, *where* it was taken from in the vagina, and the presence of vaginal infection such as monilia (thrush). Bleeding, recent intercourse and even the taking of other drugs can also affect the smear, while there is the additional problem of variation in the response of ageing tissues. Biochemical assay methods may reveal quite high levels of oestrogen in the blood, while response of the cells of the vagina may be poor and only give a low Maturation Index.

Another variable to further confuse the issue is the different interpretation of smears by different technicians, when slides have to be sent away to outside laboratories.

It is small wonder that in his excellent book *The Ageless Woman*, gynaecologist, Sherwin Kaufman, insists 'Smears are not a dependable measure of the absolute level of oestrogen in the body, especially when a single test is made'. Dr Kaufman goes on to deplore women asking to have their 'oestrogen level' checked as though it were oil for an engine, and the female tendency to confuse oestrogen levels with sex appeal. He also insists that doctors must treat the woman and not the smear, though he does concede that serial smears, as opposed to single smears, may have diagnostic value.

The test itself is painless, takes only a few seconds and can be done by any qualified doctor. It can be done, and usually is in the States, at the same time as a routine check for malignancy.

While the malignancy test requires a smear taken from the head of the cervix at the top of the vagina, the Maturation Index requires a few cells from the lateral wall of the upper third of the vagina.

Because oestrogen levels vary for each woman throughout her cycle, it is usual to take a smear at or about midcycle (fifteenth day from the start of the last period) and this applies whether a woman is menstruating, or whether she is on an induced cycle through hormone replacement or the contraceptive pill. For others who have ceased menstruation and not yet started replacement therapy, obviously there is no existing cycle to be considered, and although oestrogen levels may be low, they do still fluctuate, so that a single smear cannot always be considered totally conclusive.

Doctors specializing in HRT on both sides of the Atlantic

usually take the smear, prepare the slide and assess the ratio of cells under the microscope themselves with no delay involved. Others less familiar with the process, or not equipped for the work, must send the smear to a cytologist.

Two women whom I met in New York, gave me examples of this Maturation Index in their own cases. One was Mrs Mildred Capuro, who was aged forty-nine when I met her in 1972, but as with so many women on HRT looked very much younger. She told me she was lucky enough to have been under a doctor who believed in oestrogen replacement, so as a matter of course long before the menopause started, he had instituted vaginal smears whenever she had her routine check for malignancy. She and her doctor, therefore, knew that her normal Maturation Index was the classic, 85-15-0.

As it happened, Mrs Capuro had to have a hysterectomy, but at least she was lucky in getting immediate replacement therapy. She explained,

Within 24 hours of surgery I felt depressed and terribly weepy. It was not post-surgery 'blues', because as soon as my doctor gave me a large dose of oestrogen, these symptoms entirely disappeared.

After that I was stabilised on a forty-two day-cycle with natural oestrogen and have felt just fine. At one point a few years ago, because of a virus illness, I was taken for a while off all medication. My gynaecologist agreed we should respect this other doctor's wishes, and we both felt it would be an interesting test.

During a period of about four to six weeks I gradually sensed all the symptoms of the menopause, hot flushes, restlessness, sleeplessness and irritability. But then I was allowed back on oestrogen and gradually the depression and everything cleared up. Since, I have felt so full of energy and so well that I run my home and do a job five days a week as well, which I thoroughly enjoy.

The long forty-two-day cycle is less often prescribed by doctors these days, but twenty-eight days or thirty-five days is very common for older patients, as it is obviously more convenient to have a longer interval between any withdrawal bleeding, which, if it occurs, will come during the week off medication at the end of each cycle.

Eleanor Wilson, sister-in-law of gynaecologist Robert Wilson, explained how this had worked for her.

When my oestrogen levels suddenly dropped I felt terrible. My periods were still regular and only the Maturation Index revealed what was happening, with the ratio of mature cells falling from my usual seventy-five right down to five. I was put on natural oestrogen on a twenty-one-day cycle, then five years ago at the age of fifty, I switched to a forty-two-day cycle, which means menstruating only every six weeks. Even this can be adjusted to fit in with holidays or special occasions by stopping the tablets earlier or taking them a little longer. This method has such flexibility that it is really very little inconvenience. I know I am not young, but I still feel young, female and functioning.

Despite Eleanor Wilson's own disclaimer about being young, she was a striking example of 'looking young', still retaining the lithe figure of a dancer, which she had been before marriage.

The extended cycle has obvious advantages for a woman with an intact uterus, as it reduces the incidence of withdrawal bleeding. Even so, Eleanor Wilson's readiness to accept this controlled bleeding is by no means shared by all women. In fact, it is women's individual attitude towards menstruation which can be the determining factor in deciding the type and regimen of hormone therapy to be used.

In general terms, I have found a woman who goes on HRT right at the onset of the menopause, or even very soon after her final menstrual period, is more willing to accept continuation or renewal of bleeding than a woman who may have had a gap of several years since her periods ended. Once out of the habit of bothering with sanitary towels etc., there is a natural reluctance to start all over again.

One marvellous woman of seventy-plus, who had willingly accepted menstruation for years for the sake of feeling well and keeping young, confided that she had eventually become embarrassed about buying sanitary towels at her age. She told me, 'I pretend now that they are for my daughter, and I vary the stores I buy them from. I really think I may ask my doctor to change the therapy, because I know it is possible to have oestrogen without bleeding.'

For the many women who totally refuse to re-start menstruation, it is possible to institute oestrogen replacement at a level which eliminates symptoms but does not produce bleeding. A certain amount of trial and error is involved in finding the optimum dosage. Some doctors start fairly high to knock out the symptoms, then reduce the dosage to the lowest level at which the patient continues to be symptom-free.

Other doctors start at a low level and increase the dosage to the point at which bleeding occurs, then back-track to a level just below this. There is today a growing body of medical opinion which believes oestrogen therapy should not be designed to produce withdrawal bleeding, and in general it seems to me there is a trend toward these lower dosage techniques.

At the same time there are also many doctors who argue that such low dosages may not be sufficient to achieve full replacement and confer full protection, particularly against osteoporosis. There are also many women, and I have met them both in Britain and America, who positively welcome continuation of their cyclic life-rhythm.

One British woman told me, 'I think of my body as a machine which needs servicing. HRT is part of that servicing and it keeps my body working properly and, as it were, firing on all cylinders.'

Mrs Elizabeth Vann, whose case-history recounted earlier included such extremely good cosmetic effects on HRT, put her reaction to menstruating again more simply. She said, 'It's not a question of putting up with it again, I actually welcome it. It makes me feel young and normal.'

However, what may feel normal in the fifties may feel absurd in the seventies, and so many women as they get older ask their doctors to lower the dosage and cut out progesterone to preclude bleeding.

For those women who have had a surgical menopause, of course, the 'to bleed or not to bleed' dilemma does not arise. Without a uterus there is no such complication and oestrogen alone usually produces excellent results. As one doctor put it to me, 'These women have the best of both worlds, all the advantages of HRT at proper dosage and no complication with bleeding.'

Where the uterus is intact and where the patient is prepared to accept menstruation, there is a large body of influential medical opinion which believes the combined hormone therapy, oestrogen plus progesterone, with disciplined, induced withdrawal bleeding is desirable.

The great value of using the other female sex hormone, progesterone, alongside oestrogen over the last five to seven days of each cycle, is that this ensures orderly and regular shedding of the endometrium, within three days of stopping both pills.

This regular and expected bleeding eliminates the risk of breakthrough bleeding or spotting, which can sometimes occur in mid-cycle on oestrogen alone. But some doctors, like pioneer Robert Wilson, also insist that the regular periodic shedding of the endometrium has value in itself, lessening the risk of endometrial cancer by sloughing off unhealthy cells. Dr Wilson also argued strongly that progesterone has its own valuable part to play in the body economy, particularly in restoring normal pituitary function.[1]

While many doctors might not agree with these contentions, they would not dispute Dr Wilson's main argument for use of progesterone, that it serves to prevent over-stimulation of breasts and endometrium, which even the pill-free week cannot sometimes avoid on oestrogen alone.

Sir John Peel is a firm advocate of the combined therapy. He explained,

No one should use oestrogen alone and without interruption day in and day out. Prolonged and continuous over-stimulation of the endometrium can be a factor in producing endometrial cancer. The important rule in oestrogen replacement therapy is that it must be intermittent and I believe the combination with a progestagen is a safer system.

Sir John went on to point out that where the dosage of oestrogen necessary to control symptoms did *not* cause withdrawal or break-through bleeding, obviously there was no over-stimulation and so no necessity for progesterone. Even more obviously where there was no uterus, no problems could arise, so that a progestogen is not necessary after a hysterectomy.

Apart from this protection against over-stimulation and hyperplasia which progesterone affords, it is the disciplining of the bleeding into a regular pattern which is so valuable. Unexpected bleeding always requires investigation, as it can

D

be a sign of malignancy, and obviously frequent checks of this kind must be inconvenient for both doctor and patient.

In his book Dr Kaufman mentions the happy compromise he sometimes uses of simply inducing a shedding of the uterine lining by use of a progesterone at the end of the cycle just once or twice a year, which is enough to obviate breakthrough bleeding in most women.

Though views on the use of progesterone are somewhat divided, most doctors are agreed on the necessity for cyclic administration of oestrogen. The regular interruption of tissue stimulation is vital to avoiding over-stimulation or excessive bleeding.

It is interesting that even with hysterectomized patients, where there is no uterus, the cyclic scheme is still usually adopted, partly to guard against over-stimulation of breasts, but also because fluctuating oestrogen levels are an integral part of the normal female hormone system.

So there is a wide choice of methods and regimens, and although this may seem confusing to the lay reader, there are advantages in having different variations and techniques, so that the therapy can be tailored to individual needs and individual chemistry.

But the basic concept remains the same – the replacement of missing oestrogen – the remedy of a deficiency state.

11. The choice of oestrogens

As well as a choice of techniques and regimens, there is also, of course, a choice of oestrogens. Although so far throughout this book reference has been made to 'oestrogen', as though it were one single substance, in fact there is a whole family of these hormones secreted by the ovaries during their functioning life.

Although it was only at the beginning of this century that the hormonal nature of ovarian control of reproduction was established, and only in the 1920s that female sex hormones themselves were discovered in the urine of menstruating and pregnant women, ancient remedies were often based on placental material which is rich in oestrogen and on urine which also contains sex hormones.

The use of human placenta was first mentioned in a Chinese pharmacopoeia of AD 725, but may go back even further. Certainly by the fourteenth century it was commonly prescribed in China for all forms of debility including sexual weakness. One Chinese doctor of that period wrote,

I have often used it and obtained perfect results, especially in female patients. The merit of the placenta is chiefly to increase the efficiency of the Yin force in the body, including sexual function. It always seems to give good results. If one takes it for a long time it improves the hearing, brightens the eyes, keeps the hair and beard black, increases longevity, and indeed has such merit that it can overcome the natural process of ageing.

Even more remarkable than the unwitting use so long ago of oestrogen from the placenta, was the development of medieval Chinese medicine to include fractionation of urine, yielding end-products which quite certainly included both androgens and oestrogens.

The use of urine in the ancient medicine of many nations was written off in modern times as useless and disgusting, until the classical discovery of S. Ascheim and B. Zondek in 1927 of the presence of large amounts of sex hormones in pregnancy urine, and the subsequent discovery that the urine of all animals, but especially that of the mare, contains these substances. The horse in fact has been described as a remarkable oestrogen factory, and the pregnant mare excretes over 100 mg. daily.

Many of the family of naturally occurring oestrogens can be successfully synthesized in the laboratory, sometimes modified slightly in structure by linking with a salt. Examples include piperazine oestrone sulphate (Harmogen) which is proving a useful oestrogen for replacement therapy, and estradiol valerate (Progynova) introduced in the U.K. in 1975.

A sharp distinction should be made between such man-made versions of naturally occurring oestrogens, and those correctly termed 'synthetic oestrogens', such as stilbestrol and dienstrol. These are entirely artificial both in chemical and molecular structure, do not occur in nature and are essentially foreign to the human body.

These truly synthetic oestrogens are merely substances which possess oestrogenic-like properties, and many have been developed specifically as the basis of the contraceptive pill and for its distinctly *unnatural* task of maintaining a permanent state of infertility. For this purpose they are extremely effective.

They do, however, have certain side-effects and hazards, in particular an effect on blood-clotting potential with slightly increased thrombosis risk. With the wide choice of naturally-occurring oestrogens now available and where no contraceptive purpose is required, it seems outdated and outmoded to still prescribe synthetic oestrogens for treatment of the menopause.

An exception to this might prove to be with the sophisticated sequential concept of a preparation like Mestranol, when varied doses of the same synthetic oestrogen are given in a carefully calculated and prescribed sequence. Over the last thirteen days, the oestrogen is also combined with a progesterone, so that the body's own pre-menopause pattern of rise and fall in sex hormone levels is closely simulated. This was the technique used in the HRT clinic at Birmingham Women's Hospital, with the satisfactory and interesting results already reported.[1]

Letters from many women and conversations with many doctors make it clear, however, that other synthetic oestrogens, particularly stilbestrol, are still used far too often to relieve menopause symptoms instead of the safer naturally occurring oestrogens. It is obvious that some family doctors do not even appreciate the distinction between synthetic and naturally occurring oestrogens, and have missed the important research reports strongly indicating the latter are free from thrombosis risk.

I hasten to add that it is not difficult to sympathize with over-worked GP's who simply do not have time to keep up with the vast out-pourings of medical literature. It is less easy to sympathize with those who huff and puff about there being no such literature on Hormone Replacement. In fact the bibliography at the back of just one booklet sent by one drug company to all doctors, lists 114 papers and research sources.

From personal experience I can vouch for familiarity with hundreds more, as the piles of papers stacked on my desk bear witness. The writer of one such paper made a wry comment about doctors who grumble there is no HRT literature. He said, 'Maybe their definition of literature is what they read, not what is written.'

Natural conjugated oestrogen (Premarin), most commonly used to treat the menopause, even today is refined direct from the urine of pregnant mares. It contains the whole range of oestrogens which the body before the menopause both produces and responds to. This multiple-oestrogen content, is the reason for some doctors' preference, as they believe it should ensure wider application and relief of symptoms.

On the first television programme ever done on Hormone Replacement Therapy in the UK, which I presented for Associated Television's enterprising *Women Today*, the young gynaecologist who had been invited to oppose the concept, opened his spirited attack by scoffing at the notion of equine oestrogen as 'natural'. 'Natural to what?' he asked, 'natural to horses?'

It was a fair enough debating point, and obviously the ideal oestrogen for the ideal replacement therapy would be *human* conjugated oestrogen. In the very early days of the therapy this was even possible, with hormone from oestrogen-rich women being donated to oestrogen-poor women, in a splendid example of the ultimate in socialized medicine.

However, with growing acceptance of the logic of HRT and

growing demand for it, sufficient supplies of human oestrogen were simply not available. Fortunately it was found that the structure of equine oestrogen so closely resembled that of human oestrogen, that women were able to metabolize it perfectly well, with no side-effects and with good relief of symptoms.

Just a few of the letters I have received, however, indicate that some women are put off by the idea of oestrogen from mares' urine, while still others are concerned in case any cruelty to the animals themselves is involved.

In fact many of our most useful drugs and hormones are prepared from ostensibly unattractive animal sources. The life-saving hormone, insulin, for example, is extracted from the pancreas of pigs. It is not the source but the success and safety of the end-product which really matters.

As to ethics and suffering to animals, this has to be seen always in the context of the human suffering it saves. Happily, to obtain conjugated oestrogen, animals have to be neither killed nor maimed. In fact the special herd of eighty thousand mares out on the Canadian Plains, who supply the 'raw material' lead something of an idyllic life. All that is required of them is doing what comes naturally and being healthily and happily pregnant.

One other group of oestrogens are useful in Hormone Replacement at the menopause. These are termed 'free oestrogens' and are simply single separate members of the oestrogen family, 'freed' and isolated from the group. Examples of these include estrone, estriol and 17B estradiol.

Where progesterone, the other female sex hormone is concerned for use in the recommended combined therapy, the choice is not so wide. Unlike naturally occurring oestrogens, the natural progesterone cannot be successfully used orally, as it is broken down by the acid of the stomach and not properly absorbed into the system.

Fortunately progesterone-like molecules (called progestagens) have been developed, which are not destroyed in this way and which are successfully absorbed to perform the normal functions of natural progesterone. What is more, they do this without harmful side-effects and in particular, with no effect on platelet behaviour and no increase of thrombosis risk.

The most widely used progestagen, both in the UK and the States is Provera, but there is also Norlutin-A known in America as Norlutate.

Dr John Burch, whom I talked to in Nashville, Tennessee, emphasized how much the wider choice of oestrogens was helping both doctor and patient. He told me,

This is the first time in history that women have been able to live out their lives without being deprived of hormones somewhere along the line. I have been using oestrogen replacement since the early 1930s, but the modern oestrogens which came along in the fifties, and in particular the natural conjugated oestrogens, have made our work so much easier and safer, with fewer side-effects.

This might be an appropriate spot to list the side-effects, which just a few women do experience on oestrogen therapy. The most common is a mild form of nausea, thought to be related to the nausea that occurs during pregnancy. The naturally-occurring oestrogens appear to give rise to this far less often than synthetic oestrogens and the tendency can be minimized by taking the pills after meals. Even where such nausea occurs, it is usually only during the first cycle, or if the oestrogen dosage is too high.

Breast tenderness and swelling also sometimes occur and women who suffer from cystic mastitis can be more prone to this. Some others may experience just a little soreness, and decreasing the dose or the addition of progesterone minimizes all these problems.

As already mentioned, irregular, unexpected bleeding is the greatest disadvantage of oestrogen therapy, but cyclic administration and the use of a progestagen disciplines this.

Sometimes weight gain and swelling may occur from water retention due to oestrogen, but again, this is more common with the synthetic oestrogens.

There may be also slight darkening of the nipples and surrounding area, and occasionally some slight pigmentation freckles on the face. Changing the brand of oestrogen can eliminate this tendency too.

Finally oestrogen naturally promotes cervical secretions, and although this is desirable and far preferable to abnormal menopausal dryness, it can sometimes be excessive, and again, this can be controlled by reducing the dosage, or adding a progestagen.

Most women will not incur any of these side-effects, but where they do the wider choice of medication now available certainly means that by selecting the correct preparation and varying the dosage and regimen, it is almost always possible to find a form of HRT to suit the individual patient.

Many studies have been done to compare the positive results achieved with various oestrogens, and even more interestingly to compare them in double-blind trials against a placebo.

A placebo (from the Latin verb, to please) is simply the name given to an inactive substance, such as chalk or water, which will pass through the body with no biological effect, but which is disguised to look like some actual medication.

The term 'double-blind' indicates that neither the patient nor the doctor is aware at the time whether the placebo or the real medication is being used, though coded records enable this to be established later when it is time to compare results.

Because someone taking a placebo *believes* it is a medicine, there is often a so-called 'placebo effect', and the patient does actually feel better – proof of the influence the mind and the thinking can have on health.

It has been fashionable in some quarters to insist that many menopause symptoms are 'only in the mind', and in such cases clearly a placebo should work just as well as an oestrogen.

In practice, however, the many double-blind studies carried out have disproved this. One done by Professor G. Lauritzen and quoted at the 1972 Geneva Workshop Conference on HRT, was fairly typical. Several hundred menopausal patients were involved, and although on the placebo the expected percentage felt better, the percentage whose complaints actually disappeared was nil. In contrast on estriol (1 mg) 68% of symptoms disappeared, and on conjugated oestrogen (1·25 mg.) 92% disappeared.[2]

One would hope that this sort of result would have disposed for ever of the belief long-cherished by some men (and regrettably by some doctors) that menopause symptoms are largely psychological, a miserable nervous reaction induced in middle-aged women by the prospect of loss of fertility and loss of youth.

Where a woman's life, her interests and her sense of identity and importance have centred exclusively around either her fertility or her physical beauty, it is true the loss of these may well aggravate the menopause and other problems of ageing.

But basically menopause problems are not psychological – they are physiological and can be pathological – they result from the deficiency of oestrogen and they respond to treatment with oestrogen. They do not respond to chalk coated with sugar.

12. The implant technique

So far this book has looked only at the use of the female sex hormones, oestrogen and progesterone, in replacement therapy. But sometimes the male sex hormone, testosterone, may also have a place in the complicated hormonal picture.

Again, although HRT is most commonly achieved through tablets taken by mouth, which permits easy adjustment of dosage, oestrogen, progesterone and testosterone may instead on occasions be 'implanted' under the skin, in the form of pellets, which give a slow, continuous release of hormones over many months.

It was on my second visit to the United States in a private clinic in Augusta, Georgia, that I saw the implant system used for the first time. As my research had progressed and I had read more and more medical literature on the menopause and on replacement therapy, it had become clear that there was one doctor in America whom I had to see – that was Robert Greenblatt, Professor of Endocrinology at the Medical College of Georgia.

Not only was Dr Greenblatt one of the top endocrinologists in the world, and the man who for eighteen successive years had contributed the section on endocrinology to the year book of the *Encyclopaedia Britannica*, but he was also a top gynaecologist and pathologist. The combination of these disciplines had led him to do major work on infertility, where his development of the drug, Clomiphene, had brought him a crop of gold and silver medals, and most recently the French Order of Chevalier of the Legion of Honour.

But in addition to this, Robert Greenblatt had also for many years been a leading exponent and advocate of hormone replacement at the menopause, and my visit to Augusta was timed to coincide with a conference on the Management of Ageing, arranged at the University under his auspices as President of the prestigious American Geriatric Society.

With doctors flying in from all over America, with his own house-guests and his own lectures scheduled, I was a little dubious about how much time he would manage to spare me. I need not have worried. On my first morning he joined me with other doctors for breakfast at my hotel before 8.30 a.m., so that we could talk before the official programme started. This sort of energy and dynamism was just as evident in his approach to HRT, and spilled over into the charisma from which his patients clearly drew immense confidence.

His position regarding HRT was very simple.

A basic premise in endocrinology is to restore hormonal balance [he explained]. Oestrogen deficit after the menopause should be relieved just as much as thyroidal, pancreatic or andrenal deficits, and it should be replaced by oestrogen, not by homespun psychology or tranquillisers. How can either of these be expected to arrest a deteriorating metabolic milieu? And why should barbiturates, bromides and tranquillisers, so foreign to the human organism, be preferable to natural oestrogen?

Dr Greenblatt estimates that 75% of women become acutely oestrogen-deficient within a few years of the menopause, and believes HRT should be offered to every woman with symptoms and even to those without, if an oestrogen deficit is present. In particular he insists that even in the absence of any other symptoms, the presence of osteoporosis is sufficient reason to initiate therapy with small doses of oestrogen (along with increased calcium and protein intake and exercise) for the rest of the patient's lifetime. He told me, 'Oestrogens appear to apply a brake to the parathyroids' capacity to stimulate bone resorption, and in severe osteoporosis, oestrogens protect by minimizing further skeletal deterioration and collapse of vertebrae.'

For oral HRT, Dr Greenblatt uses the natural conjugated oestrogen, Premarin, but where a patient is prepared to accept menstruation he prescribes *continuous* administration. But he still produces a cyclic effect and regular shedding by interposing a progestagen (Provera or Norlutate) alongside the oestrogen for five to seven days in each month.

Like Sir John Peel, he is convinced about the importance of using progesterone. He insisted,

Where you are going to give oestrogen in full replacement dosage to a woman with an intact uterus, there should be a functioning, secreting endometrium. Oestrogens alone can produce complications such as painful breasts, weight gain, irregular bleeding and hyperplasia (abnormal thickening of normal tissue). All this is avoided and bleeding disciplined with the use of a progestagen, and with such a safeguard, I believe it is correct to keep the oestrogen continuous to avoid recurrence of symptoms and increased resorption of bone, that otherwise would occur during the week when oestrogen is withdrawn.

Where patients are unable to accept monthly bleeding, Dr Greenblatt prescribes a lower dosage of natural oestrogen (usually ·625 mg.) which is taken daily from Monday to Friday, with Saturday and Sunday off in each week. This system of short cycles is designed to avoid any breakthrough bleeding or withdrawal bleeding.

But because so many patients come to him from great distances, flying in from as far away as Rhodesia, Canada San Francisco and even South Africa, Dr Greenblatt makes considerable use of the implant technique. He explained to me, 'Sometimes these patients come from areas where there is no local doctor able to supervise Hormone Replacement. The implant method confers six months' trouble-free replacement, and the slow release mechanism is particularly effective.'[1]

On my second day in Augusta, I was given the chance to judge this for myself. Suitably clad in a white coat, and with the permission of each patient, I took my place with the medical team working with Dr Greenblatt at one of his private clinic sessions.

On that day there was the usual broad spectrum of problems a gynaecologist and endocrinologist must deal with. In particular there were many young women with infertility problems, and I was lucky enough to witness the happiness of one girl and her husband, when they learned that after a course of Clomiphene the on-the-spot pregnancy test and examination confirmed conception. It was a great moment for us all.

As well as infertility, there were cases of frigidity also responding well to hormone treatment, and there were several young patients being treated for problems of growth.

However, it was the varied crop of menopausal cases, both

surgical and natural, which were of special interest to me. As it happened on that particular day, they were all on return visits, and so the usual six-monthly check-up was done, with internal examination and smear tests. The slides were examined by Dr Greenblatt there and then under the microscope to confirm the level of replacement was correct and that the vaginal mucosa was healthy. Once this was established, a repeat implant was done.

This proved a very minor surgical procedure and quite painless. First a shot of local anaesthetic was injected into the lower abdomen, and then immediately a small metal tube was inserted in the same area, down which the appropriate hormone pellets were introduced. The tube was withdrawn, a piece of sticking-plaster applied and that was that. It took only a few seconds, though the effect would last for up to six months.

In some cases along with the oestrogen pellet or pellets (each 25 mg. of pure estradiol), Dr Greenblatt also inserted a pellet or pellets of male testosterone (75 mg.) and he explained,

I have found the administration of testosterone along with the oestrogen enhances the benefit, frequently in eliminating depression while improving energy and sex drive. There is also often considerable improvement in any arthritic condition, but the unexpected bonus has been in relief of migraine-type headaches. While oral HRT relieves these in approximately 40% of cases, the ratio rises to about 80% with the implant system.

I asked Dr Greenblatt about the risk of virilizing effects, such as facial hair-growth and deepening voice which has been associated with the use of male sex hormones by women. He was reassuring about this and told me,

The excessive use of testosterone in the past has given rise to fears about this and to some condemnation of doctors who prescribe it. As much as 25 mg. of testosterone propionate was sometimes prescribed per week for up to six months, which meant a woman was taking in all 600 mg. over the period. But with the implant method, a pellet only contains 75 mg., and this is released slowly over the same length of time, adding up to only one-eighth of that dose. Even where two pellets are required, it is still only one-quarter of the dose.

From his thirty-five years' experience, Robert Greenblatt estimates only between 5% and 10% of women may show some slight virilizing effects, and then it is usually only a small increase in facial hair. If this does happen, such patients have the option of discontinuing the testosterone, when the hair growth usually recedes. But Dr Greenblatt told me that most of the few women affected prefer to still continue the treatment because they feel so well on the combined therapy. He explained, 'They are often women, who after surgical or natural menopause, have suffered almost total loss of libido, which this treatment has restored. The male sex hormone does not change the direction of sex drive, but it does intensify the response.'

Dr Greenblatt made the point that for many women oestrogen replacement alone is enough to restore sexual feeling.

It eliminates dryness, makes the vaginal mucosa softer and more succulent and ensures proper lubrication, and this all means that sexual relations become easier and more enjoyable. This in itself brings a marked improvement in response. But where oestrogen alone fails to achieve this, then testosterone should be added. It can also be given orally in the form of methyltestosterone at 2·5 mg. per day over short periods. Again if virilizing reactions start to occur, it is simple to discontinue treatment.

Only one out of the six patients I saw and talked to, who were having testosterone implants, had developed a facial hair problem. She was an attractive brunette of about thirty-five, who had had her ovaries removed and who admitted she had always been a slightly 'hairy' type. Although Dr Greenblatt did suggest she might like to forgo just one of her testosterone pellets, she refused, 'My husband is happy the way things are,' she explained. 'We have a great sex life and I can get the hair growth dealt with quite easily.'

Because I had already met so many women on oral HRT, I chose particularly to talk to those receiving implants. Another one was Gail McCuan, aged twenty-seven from South Carolina, who had had both ovaries removed some years before.

Pellets of oestrogen and testosterone were implanted even before my operation so I never suffered any drastic symptoms afterwards.

But I soon notice when the action of the implants begins to decline toward the end of each six-month period. Then I get tired and depressed and have no sexual response. But within a day or two of the new implants, I am back to normal and feeling fine.

Another patient who talked to me very frankly was Mrs Leonora Holtzman, who had flown in from Miami, Florida. Fifty years old, blonde and attractive, she looked far too young to have two grown-up children and four grandchildren. She told me,

After a hysterectomy at the age of forty-one, I had a terrible time. I had fearful sweats every night and awful depression. The worst part for me was my inability to cope with life. At that time my children were giving me a lot of problems, and when I finally flew to Georgia to see Dr Greenblatt that first time, I remember telling my husband that if this doctor could not help me, I would not come home . . . and I meant it. I was really at the end of my tether. My doctor back home had told me that I needed a psychiatrist and I had begun to believe him. But the hormone replacement revolutionized my life. I've been coming back ever since for my two testosterone and one oestrogen pellets. With me they only last four months, probably because I lead such an energetic life. I feel so well and full of energy now, that I am even tackling the job of bringing up my seven-year-old grandson.

Mrs Evelyne Thorpe from Athens, Georgia, was another patient who had been on implants for ten years, in her case to counteract a severe natural menopause. Aged fifty-six and a widow, she received no testosterone just two oestrogen pellets. She told me,

Before treatment I suffered terribly from hot flushes and night sweats that left me drenching wet. After the first implant the symptoms disappeared completely. Now, even if I didn't have my next appointment fixed, I'd know when the six months was up, because I begin to feel exhausted and that is the signal that the implant is running out. Within seven days of having the new implant I feel energetic and well again.

Although there could be no doubt about the effectiveness of the implant system, there were some obvious disadvantages. The first was the cost – each batch of implants costs seventy-five dollars, which even by American standards put implant replacement therapy into the category of privileged medicine. But apart from the cost, there is the fact that the dosage cannot be so easily adjusted or so swiftly changed as with oral medication, though implants can be recovered and removed if this is really necessary for any reason. To avoid problems such as excessive bleeding, the sort of meticulous biochemical investigation carried out by Robert Greenblatt is essential.

Of course the implant system of HRT is also used outside America, and was pioneered in the UK by London gynaecologist, Mr E. Schleyer-Saunders. In 1973 in the *South African Journal of Obstetrics and Gynaecology*, Mr Schleyer-Saunders published the results of a study he had carried out on a series of one thousand patients, all of whom he had treated with implants. The oestrogen used was also estradiol, with dosages varying between 15 and 25 mg., according to the oestrogen deficiency determined from vaginal smears. In some cases 50 mg. of progesterone and 25 mg. testosterone was also administered as pellets.

Relief of symptoms, particularly flushes and vaginal atrophy, was good and Mr Schleyer-Saunders noted while bleeding occurred in 20% of cases treated with oestrogen implant alone, this was reduced to only 5% with the combined use of oestrogen, progesterone and testosterone.

In line with other studies on *oral* HRT, it was also found in this implant study that the incidence of cancer was somewhat lower than would generally be expected in women of the same age in the general population. No cases of venous thrombosis or embolism had been observed in the series at all.[2]

In Britain too the present cost of implant Hormone Replacement tends to make it largely privileged medicine, and it is usually prescribed privately. The exception is the growing use of implants at the actual time of removal of ovaries, which is being done more and more in NHS hospitals.

In the past British gynaecologists did not much favour the idea of immediate oestrogen replacement at the time of surgery, because of what they considered to be the added thrombosis risk. But with the increased use of *natural* oestrogens, or with implants which involve only low dosage release of the hormone, fewer surgeons still raise this objection and more and more women now are benefiting from this immediate replacement technique.

One hospital leading the way in this is the John Radcliffe Hospital, Oxford, and a report on this aspect of their work was given at the 20th British Congress of Obstetrics and Gynaecology, which I attended in 1974 in London. Details were presented of a comparison carried out of two groups of patients after bilaterial oophorectomy. Each patient in one group had received an implant of 100 mg. estradiol 17B (Organon) at the time of the operation. Women in the smaller group had received no implants. There was a striking difference in their subsequent experience.

Eleven of the fourteen patients in the small group with no implants developed severe flushes, and five of them required oestrogen therapy. None of the twenty-three patients with an implant, seen in the first fifteen months after surgery, had hot flushes at all. Only one of another fifteen patients with implants seen between sixteen and twenty-four months after surgery had developed mild flushes, as had two out of four patients examined after twenty-four months. All three of these women dated the onset of flushes to approximately eighteen months after the operation, indicating these particular implants as effective for between one-and-a-half and two years.[3]

Advocates of the implant system point out that the concentration of hormones required is only about one-third of the dose needed by the oral route, and also that implants avoid any untoward gastric or intestinal side-effects, which can sometimes occur with hormone tablets taken by mouth. They claim also that psychologically the patient is not continuously reminded of her condition by having to adopt a daily pill routine.

This avoidance of the need for daily tablet taking can certainly be an advantage where the patient is either not sufficiently motivated to remember, or sometimes is simply incapable of remembering. But there are advantages too for women whose jobs involve a lot of travelling, difficult hours or other pressures which interfere with a set routine.

This applies very much to women in show business, who are obvious candidates for HRT anyway, as they depend so much on appearance and vitality, not just for personal success but for professional survival.

Films, television and stage work make tremendous demands

both physically and mentally, and no middle-aged actress can afford to put a production or her own career in hazard by allowing herself to fall victim to hot flushes, lack of memory or lack of energy, all of which are so often part of the menopause.

Although a great many stars are on HRT, particularly in America, they are not over-keen to talk about it, rather in the same way that they avoid admitting to face-lifts or cosmetic surgery. Admitting that you are combating any form of ageing, is tantamount to admitting that you *are* ageing.

One pleasantly forthright star, who has no such inhibitions and who was only too happy to tell me she had used Premarin for some years, was Canadian-born, Barbara Kelly. She looks young enough to persuade anyone that HRT works, as does Jean Kent, another star willing to talk about it.

Jean favours the implant system, and her 1974 West End appearance playing the lead in *No sex please, we're British* confirmed her still considerable verve and attraction.

She is known both sides of the Atlantic for films such as *The Browning Version* and *Woman in Question,* and television plays such as *Vanity Fair* and *A Night with Mrs De Tanka.*

Jean Kent talked frankly about her own attitude,

A woman's biology is very important in my business. This is specially true of the menopause. I was brought up very sensibly by my mother to take all these things in my stride. Menstruation occasionally involved me in severe pain, but it never stopped me working. The main trouble is that it affects the voice. An opera singer never sings at that time – her programme is always arranged to avoid that. When I was having singing lessons, my singing master always had to know about this, because it changed the quality of the voice, particularly on the first day.

Then in filming I might ask the camera-man to avoid close-ups on those days. But the menopause can be even more of a problem. Once the ovaries start to pack up and you are no longer fertile, there's no doubt that nature loses interest in keeping you attractive. Also, of course, those hot flushes can be terrible things – not to be laughed off. You feel as though you've burning coals right through your body and nothing you do will cool you down.

When it started with me I went straight to my gynaecologist and once he was convinced it really was the change of life, he put me on hormone implants.

I never believe in making a fuss, but nor do I believe in suffering unnecessarily both from a personal point of view, and of course from a professional one, if I feel my work is going to suffer too.

Acting does require good health. Television imposes long rehearsal hours, with clothes fittings often having to be done in the lunch hour because of tight schedules. Films are more leisurely during the day, but involve long hours starting in the Make-Up room at 7.00 a.m., and you still have to look as fresh at 6.00 p.m. as you did in the morning. The stage in contrast is a matter of only a few hectic hours, but these are in front of a crowded house and use up more strength to the minute than films or television put together.

HRT has certainly maintained my stamina. The implant is made under a local anaesthetic into the muscle of the buttock. It starts working at once and continually day and night like a woman's own ovaries with a slow release of hormone. The result is excellent and I can tell when I am almost due for another treatment, as I find myself getting the occasional flush and tiring more easily.

I've seen friends of mine with hot flushes so fierce that they dare not go into a store to shop, but have to get someone else to do it while they wait outside. Then others go through bouts of terrible depression. I've recommended replacement therapy to several of them and they've all benefited from it.

Although HRT by implant can cost around £40 in Britain at the moment, advocates insist the costs will come down as the system becomes more widely used.

Opponents still maintain, however, that except in a few cases where oral replacement is not well tolerated, the disadvantages of the implant method outweigh advantages. They emphasize the risk of excessive bleeding and the greater difficulty of adjusting dosage, the higher cost, and the fact that in the case of the women with an intact uterus, oestrogen-stimulation by an implant is continuous. Although this may be offset by the addition of progesterone and also by the lower dosages involved, there is no doubt more work is needed to compare the relative value of oral and implant methods. This is currently being done in a special study being carried out under Professor Philip Rhodes at St Thomas's Hospital, London.

In all aspects of HRT there are still many questions to be answered, many claims to be confirmed and a great deal still to be learned. At least the time of apathy is passed. Women are being alerted to its benefits, doctors forced to recognize its potential, and research is being undertaken which within a decade should answer most of the important outstanding questions.

13. Present problems and future hopes

When Queen Victoria was faced with reluctant doctors who objected to her insistence on the new chloroform being used to ease a royal birth, she is reputed to have royally clinched the argument with the words, '*We* are having the baby; *we* shall have the chloroform.'

Perhaps it is time, even without such royal authority, that middle-aged women wanting Hormone Replacement and faced with uncooperative doctors, tried exerting similar female firmness to insist, '*We* are having the menopause; *we* shall have Hormone Replacement.'

For the real problem facing women today in connection with HRT reflects the basic problem facing them in every sphere of life – the problem of how to enforce their equal rights, including the right to make their own vital decisions, particularly decisions concerning their own bodies.

With the increased availability of contraception and abortion, women are already winning the right to decide if and when they will have a child. Now that HRT offers the choice, and the weight of medical evidence shows it to be a safe one, women should surely also have the right to decide if and when they will have the menopause.

As we have seen it is by no means a purely selfish decision. They impose upon themselves the discipline of regular cycles of pill-taking, but in return they gain better physical, mental and emotional health which benefits not only themselves but the family and society.

So how should the woman who has decided she wants HRT set about getting it? From the hundreds of letters I receive from women who have been refused the treatment by their doctors, I can certainly confirm how *not* to set about it. Do not, as many of these rather desperate women did, sail into your doctor waving some article extolling HRT (or even this book) and demand to be put on oestrogen there and then.

Nothing is more understandably calculated to put up the back of your doctor, who is entitled to consider himself the professional adviser in the situation, with a right to form his own judgement and make his own suggestions for treatment.

There is, as every wise woman knows, far more to being a feminist (and to being a woman) than setting out to bulldoze a way through by militant aggression, even before weighing up the existence of opposition. The suffragettes in England, wonderful women though they were, actually may have set back the cause of women in that country by heroic militancy which served to both rouse and build up innate male hostility. In contrast, it is interesting to note how much easier the path of emancipation has proved for women in some eastern countries, with no such background of female militancy, where they have progressed straight from purdah to parliament (and even Premiership) with little or no opposition.

So, in the battle for HRT as in other women's battles, the first approach should be tactful. The immediate task is to establish a menopause situation that requires treatment by explaining symptoms and problems. Then, if the doctor or gynaeologist does not himself suggest HRT, obviously the time has come for you to mention it. Diplomatically indicate that you have heard about Hormone Replacement and how well it works and wish to try it. If you are still met with total unwillingness to prescribe it, or even the compromise of giving it a short-term trial, then the only course is to state firmly that you intend to get a second opinion.

Of course as more and more doctors are converted to HRT the whole problem of availability will diminish. It is already far easier to obtain than it was even three years ago. Although widely differing views on the subject still persist they do not remain static. Except in a few cases where minds are shut and positions entrenched, opinions are constantly being modified and even entirely changed in favour of HRT, as new research and findings are published, or earlier reports become more widely known.

One man to change his views on HRT was John Studd, the gynaecologist who appeared on that first television programme and made the jolly quip about equine oestrogen only being natural for horses.

That was in 1972, and it was clear then that John Studd was not only sceptical about the equine oestrogen but about the actual value of replacement therapy, which he believed to be largely unproven, except in the short-term to relieve specific menopause symptoms.

Although he gave no indication on the programme itself but stuck firmly to his opposition role, it seems he was nevertheless impressed by some of the material quoted by John Maddison, the doctor advocating the therapy in the television debate. At any rate, he subsequently checked up the various references and set about reading up other medical literature on the subject. Finally, during his next spell of leave from his NHS post, he took himself out to the States to carry out a first-hand appraisal of the work being done there in the HRT field.

As a result, since his return, John Studd (now consultant at King's College Hospital, London) has set up three HRT clinics in this country, all operating under the NHS and all concerned with long-term studies and follow-up. He has also written widely on the subject and in one article published in March, 1974, he not only expressed his own views but neatly set the current scene in British medicine. He wrote,

Regrettably, too many doctors allow patients with post-menopausal vasomotor symptoms to 'sweat out' the menopause. The treatment of the asymptomatic woman is regarded with even less enthusiasm.

Administration of oral oestrogen plays an important role in the treatment of the symptoms of the climacteric, particularly for vasomotor attacks and atrophic vaginitis. Although these are the most easily identifiable features of the climacteric symptoms, they may not be the most distressing. Some of the related emotional problems are also helped by oestrogen therapy where the vasomotor attacks produce insomnia, fatigue, forgetfulness and anxiety. Oestrogens would be a far better choice of primary therapy than the antidepressants which are so widely prescribed for post-menopausal women.

I believe that oestrogens are used far too infrequently in the management of climacteric symptoms. Women can be desperately unhappy with the combined problems of dyspareunia [painful intercourse] hot sweats and tiredness. When combined with a paranoid feeling of physical and domestic rejection, the menopause becomes a cruel emotional load which can in many cases be eased by small doses of synthetic or natural oestrogen.

The resistance of British gynaecologists to long-term oestrogen therapy reflects a belief that such therapy represents a particularly unpleasant side of North American private practice. For the unscrupulous, hormone replacement therapy has no equal as a money-spinner. Over-riding this emotive attitude is the belief that the claims have not been proven, although the side-effects of oestrogen therapy are well-known.

The principal fear that oestrogen therapy is carcinogenic is in fact illogical because, although there is a very clear relationship between functioning oestrogen-secreting ovarian tumours with endometrial carcinoma, there is no evidence whatsoever that administered oestrogens have produced this pathology. Reputable reports from oestrogen replacement studies suggest that the incidence of breast and endometrial carcinoma is very much lower in these women.

Perhaps hormone replacement therapy will be seen as a major form of preventive medicine in our enlarging geriatric population. If so, it will create a logistic problem which will need great financial resources from the National Health Service.

John Studd's article certainly pinpoints some of the very different problems inherent in the very different medical systems obtaining in the UK and in the States.

In Britain there is the fundamental question of how far HRT can and should be integrated into the Health Service, and this is bound up with the broader question of how much emphasis should be placed in future planning on the role of preventive medicine. For it is into this category that perhaps replacement therapy ideally should be fitted.

At this moment Britain is struggling to operate a National Health Service inadequately funded and staffed, within a limited economy already drained by extensive social and welfare commitments. In these circumstances, there is currently no option but to adopt a system of stern priorities. Serious illness, urgent operations and all life-and-death situations are dealt with promptly and efficiently, with expensive equipment, X-ray procedures, tests, biopsies, anaesthesia, surgery and drugs, all supplied free of charge.

In contrast less urgent cases must often wait for weeks and sometimes months for treatment under NHS, and many middle and upper income groups opt for private treatment, or join additional private insurance schemes such as BUPA (British United Provident Association). In many cases they continue with the family doctor service under NHS, but if specialist treatment is needed they obtain this privately. It is no better – it is merely quicker.

Present pressures on existing NHS services mean that currently preventive medicine gets low priority. But some forms have won well-deserved places with the NHS structure. Free contraceptive clinics, for example, and free contraception, justify themselves not only in terms of greater personal and family stability, but in aiding better economic planning. No country today can allow unchecked population growth, if the government is to budget even for present living standards, let alone for improved conditions.

Mass screening for tuberculosis coupled with modern drugs has almost wiped out that disease, and vaccinations against polio, typhoid, smallpox, diphtheria and measles are routine preventive medicine, often organized via post-natal and school clinics.

But there is strong argument for better preventive medicine and screening later in life, and the argument becomes stronger as the ratio of older people in every population continues to grow. The 1970 census in the United States showed, out of the 104 million women in the population, 27 million were fifty years or over, with each woman at fifty having the expectation of living another twenty-eight years.

The ratio in the UK is very similar and more than a quarter of all women in the developed world are post-menopausal.

The magnitude of the public health challenge this presents cannot be under-estimated, and it is already being met in most countries with a system of regular screening for cervical cancer. Unfortunately in Great Britain, despite good facilities and wide publicity, women are proving tragically reluctant to come forward for the quick and painless check-up, offered free under the NHS, which can ensure early detection and cure.

Clinics for the older woman offering a more general service, including HRT, could be one answer. One of Britain's leading woman gynaecologists, consultant at a large London hospital, told me,

Hormone replacement therapy is the indicated treatment for women, wherever there are menopause symptoms or proven oestrogen deficiency. It can bring immense benefit, but it will bring even greater benefit if it succeeds also in persuading women to have regular vaginal and cervical smears. I believe those who are at present reluctant to come forward for check-up specifically to preclude malignancy, might respond much more readily in the wider context. Women must be educated to avail themselves of these forms of preventive medicine.

Dr Greta Malmberg, the seventy-three-year-old doctor already mentioned as a long-term user of HRT, and who works in school clinics, added her own views on this. She said, 'We already have Family Planning clinics, pre-natal clinics, ante-natal clinics and school clinics. It seems to me it is time we also had special clinics for the mature woman.'

Such clinics are already coming into existence attached to the Gynaecology Departments of many hospitals in the UK, but there is still a big snag inherent in the British system for women whose own doctors refuse not only to prescribe HRT but also to refer them elsewhere.

Under the rules of the National Health Service, a referral letter is required from the GP before a patient can properly consult a specialist. In this respect Great Britain is different not only to America, but to France, Germany, Italy, Spain, and, indeed, most other countries.

So far as NHS specialist consultants and clinics are concerned this ruling is strictly enforced, but in the private sector, a direct approach from a patient is by no means always rebuffed, although the GP is usually informed subsequently of any diagnosis or treatment that has been advised. This must obviously be done, because the GP, responsible for day-to-day care of patients, must know exactly what drugs or special treatment they may be having.

But the positively feudal relationship existing in Britain between some doctors and their patients can mean even such medical liaison being seen as a threat. One woman told me, 'My doctor not only refused to consider giving me oestrogen replacement, but actually said "I forbid you to go elsewhere" when I asked to be referred. He was in a towering rage about it all and I dare not tell him I have now been privately. It will be hopeless if the gynaecologist insists on contacting him.'

It is unfortunate that the ancient mystique surrounding medicine (so necessary when doctors had little but mystique to rely upon) and the privileged position accorded doctors over the centuries as the wise men in a largely uneducated society, should be allowed to linger on in the over-autocratic attitudes of some doctors today.

Modern drugs and techniques make the preservation of medical mystique and mystery unnecessary; the higher level of general education and the proven status of women make autocracy unacceptable. Unfortunately the very nature of the Health Service almost inadvertently helps to compound both anachronisms.

It is not intended, but with hospital services in short supply and doctors' lists often full, it is a seller's market, and the buyer, the patient, is often made to feel a supplicant. Despite the high level of Health Service contributions paid during his working life, he is not always even conscious he is a 'buyer'. He tends instead to feel it is all 'free' and he really should not grumble or assert himself.

By contrast the doctor has no hesitation in asserting *himself*. In many cases where a woman has dared to go ahead and seek HRT privately against her own doctor's wishes, the retribution has been swift. One woman wrote to me in great distress,

My doctor was so furious when he found out what I had done that he told me I must find another doctor. He would no longer keep me on his list. I don't mind so much for myself because I feel I have lost faith in him since the treatment he refused to give me has got rid so entirely of the flushes and back-ache I have suffered for years. But it is awkward and embarrassing with my husband and children being registered with him.

It is an accepted credo that a patient who is not happy about diagnosis or treatment has the right to ask for a second opinion, or to be referred for specialist advice. In fact the relevant clause of the Health Service rules is not at all clear. In describing the services a doctor must give, it states that these shall include 'arranging for referring patients, as necessary, to any other services provided under the Health Service

Acts'. These embrace all forms of specialist consultation, but obviously the crux of the interpretation lies in the words 'as necessary' and *who* decides what is necessary.

As the professional in the situation, the doctor not unnaturally often feels he alone is equipped to make such a decision. But if he is already anti-HRT, this may well influence his judgement. And in relation to the menopause in particular, it can be argued that only the woman herself can really judge how necessary it is for her to obtain help and proper relief of symptoms.

In fact most women still stand in such awe of their doctors that if treatment and referral are both refused, that may be the end of the matter. Only the strongly motivated, determined and intelligent woman dares to press on, either by changing her doctor or by making a direct approach for specialist help.

In one area where a feature article of mine had drawn attention not only to the value of HRT, but to the fact that an NHS clinic was being started at one of the large hospitals in the city, many women faced with the frustration of uncooperative GPs approached the clinic direct. The clinic, eager to begin a long-term study of HRT and needing patients, accepted them.

Some of the women probably informed their doctors what they had done, unaware that it was not strictly 'ethical'. At any rate there was an immediate and vigorous protest from several GPs, who complained to their local Medical Committee. The Chairman himself visited the Professor of Obstetrics at the hospital and the clinic was completely shut down for six long weeks, while the matter was sorted out.

These dog-in-the-manger GPs were not prepared to give the women either oestrogen replacement themselves or letters of referral to a clinic, committed to the objective study of the problem. Their professional pride and feelings had been hurt when they were 'by-passed', as one of them put it, or when their patients were 'syphoned off', as another chose to describe it. In such circumstances the much vaunted 'welfare of the patient' seemed to come a poor second to other considerations.

Within the letter of the law, as laid down by NHS rulings, these doctors were right and clinic and patients wrong. Since this episode, NHS clinics have been firmly told not to accept self-referred patients, and so this leaves a socially unjust situation, with one law for the rich and one for the poor. Any woman who can afford to pay can get round the referral letter ruling via the private sector. Alternatively as she probably lives in less crowded surroundings, she will also have a better chance of changing her doctor, if she decides that is the best way of tackling the impasse.

In this event, however, she will still be faced with the associated problem of finding out which doctors or which consultants prescribe the treatment she wants, a difficult matter without the help of her own doctor.

Getting this sort of information is again made particularly hard by the rules of professional conduct obtaining in the UK. In most countries doctors are allowed to indicate any special expertise or interest on their professional plates. In Britain this is not permitted. The little 'blue-book' of the General Medical Council lays down strict rules for doctors, designed to prevent any form of advertising or publicity, which might procure them professional advantage or financial gain.

This makes it extremely difficult for television, radio, newspapers or magazines to give real practical help to women wanting to know where to obtain HRT. Not only may names of doctors not be given over the air or published, but may not even be given in the separate private replies sent to the hundreds who furnish stamped, addressed envelopes. One very well-known clergyman was driven to write indignantly on behalf of a whole group of ladies in his parish, frustrated in their efforts to obtain HRT. Canon Norman Power, the vicar of Ladywood, Birmingham wrote,

My wife and many friends were interested in the two excellent programmes you presented on oestrogen therapy. These ladies wrote to various members of the panel and the producer, in each case receiving a letter advising them to 'consult their own doctor'. With their own doctors as hostile and unsympathetic as the worst described on your programme, what is the use of that sort of advice?

Please do not leave it there. It is unfair to dangle a dream of better health and vitality without giving the means of achievement. HRT should not be reserved just for the glamorous women who appear on your programme.

Touché. But unfortunately the complicated clauses of the relevant section VIII cover notices or announcements circulated or made public in connection with a doctor's practice and also the use of his name in articles, interviews, broadcasts, television programmes or books, where this might result in patients coming to him.

Again these rather sweeping regulations manage to be both intimidating and at the same time vague of interpretation. Unfortunately rulings on them can often only be obtained in retrospect, when the offence, if it is one, will have been committed, rather than in advance when it might be prevented.

All this has been highlighted for me over the last few years, when I have been writing features on HRT and also presenting radio and television programmes. Some of the situations provoked appear, to the lay mind at least, somewhat bizarre.

For example, some doctors give permission for their names to be used alongside quotes which make it crystal clear they approve of and prescribe HRT. Others, regardless of their views, insist that they must remain anonymous, sometimes even when they are engaged full-time in NHS work and could not possibly profit personally from the publicity.

On television the position can be particularly absurd. It is clear that doctors appearing will be recognized by patients, professional colleagues, friends (and for that matter by enemies too). Despite this, many feel the blue-book ruling prevents them allowing their names to be used. Others, participating in the same programme, have no such inhibitions, and this is just as well. Pity the poor interviewer faced with a medley of medics, *all* of whom she must only address as 'doctor'. The end result would be a programme in which no one, including the viewer, knew whom was being addressed or who was talking.

But far more important than such relatively minor inconvenience, is the fact that in all this concern about fair practice, no one seems concerned about fair practice for the patient. For whatever good and worthy reasons the rules on advertising were devised, they have the side-effect of blocking communication and of setting up barriers which prevent the patient making contact with the right specialist, unless she has the backing of her own doctor. This can have the effect of reducing the compassion and effectiveness of what, despite shortage of funds, must be acknowledged the finest Health Service in the world.

The Chairman of the local Medical Committee in England's second city of Birmingham, Dr Lew Lloyd, defended the existing system. He explained to me,

Good relations between doctor and consultant are essential to the good medical care of the patient, and the system of referral letters is vital. Most doctors, I am sure, consider their patient's wishes regarding referral, and more than thirty years of practice has certainly convinced me that it is not wise to frustrate a patient in these matters. Goodwill and rapport between doctor and patient is of first importance.

If this enlightened attitude were universal, obviously there would be no problem. But human nature being what it is, some doctors are obstinate and uncompromising, some patients irritating and less than tactful. It is never wise to *demand* HRT; it can be undiplomatic unless you know your doctor well, to wave articles extolling HRT under his nose. Women do have a right to indicate that they know such a therapy exists and is being widely used by gynaecologists of the highest standing. And, if they have clear menopausal symptoms, they have the right to ask to be allowed to try it.

Of course, as more and more doctors and gynaecologists are converted to the value of HRT and reassured about its long-term safety, the problem of getting treatment will diminish. But meanwhile there is a case for NHS Menopausal Clinics to be open to women *without* referral, in the same way as Family Planning Clinics are, providing their GPs are notified if treatment is considered to be needed.

An alternative would be some form of referral centres, perhaps even utilizing the network of Family Planning Clinics that already exist. Doctors at FP clinics could not perhaps be expected to add to their work-load by actually supervising hormone therapy, but they could have lists of HRT centres or hospitals where it can be obtained, and put women in touch with the nearest.

If it were practical, there is an argument for FP clinics in time being asked to extend their work to cover HRT. With their terms of reference already covering advice on sexual problems, they do get a number of menopausal women asking for help when vaginal atrophy starts to make intercourse painful. Also, patients who have attended over the years for contraception, inevitably run into the tricky period with the onset of the menopause when sometimes a skilful combination of HRT and the contraceptive pill is required. The 'change' is a time when for most women it is above all vital to prevent conception, and when unfortunately irregular menstruation increases anxiety and fear of pregnancy. Low dose contraceptive pills, with some additional natural oestrogen to top up declining hormone levels, can be the answer to regularize periods, give safe contraception and at the same time eliminate early menopausal problems.

The advantages of the American medical set-up, with regard to HRT and in more general terms, seem mainly confined to those lucky enough to possess a good deal of money, or incomes sufficient to permit adequate private health insurance cover. In either of these cases, the system of private medical practice permits the great boon of freedom of choice, not just in selecting *a* doctor, but in selecting *the* doctor for the job.

With no compulsory referral or registration, and with professional plates clearly indicating specialist interest and knowledge, there is no problem for the American woman in finding a doctor or gynaecologist to prescribe replacement therapy, providing she can pay for it or is covered for it by her medical insurance.

Even under the insurance schemes which most middle-income Americans use, medical treatment remains on the same private basis, with complete freedom of choice in regard to doctors. The bill is presented to the patient by the doctor or hospital, and recovered later in total or in part, depending on the scale and terms of the patient's insurance.

Most women get their Hormone Replacement Therapy in this way, but it is a different matter for the very poor. Those on social welfare do qualify for free medical care, but how often this would include something like HRT varies from State to State, hospital to hospital and even doctor to doctor. Whereas urgent medical treatment is provided and the bill taken care of by the State, a therapy more concerned with the quality of life than preservation of life is less likely to be supplied.

Between the very poor on social welfare and qualifying for free medical services, and the middle-income group who wisely go in for medical insurance, there is also a strata of people on low incomes, who would not qualify for free medical treatment and who are inclined to gamble on continuing good health, because they cannot or will not budget for insurance payments. Their predicament highlights the disadvantage of voluntary rather than compulsory health insurance, because without spare money and without insurance cover, medical help is sometimes sought too little and too late.

With compulsory health insurance reputed to be only just around the corner for America, it is to be hoped a way can be found of closing the gaps in medical care for all, while retaining the valuable freedom of choice.

Meanwhile, as mentioned earlier, the American system like any other system of private medicine does involve some pressure on the doctor to comply with the patient's wishes. Otherwise both patient and fee simply go elsewhere.

If a doctor has real grounds for believing the treatment a patient wants is actually wrong or harmful, he is faced with a choice between maintaining his professional integrity or his bank account.

On the question of the risk of exploitation of the patient by the doctor, which British medicine appears to see as the great danger of a purely private medical system, the opportunity for this most certainly exists. I can only say in my own admittedly limited experience of American medicine, I did not find evidence of it being very widespread.

Obviously in all countries and all systems, there will always be some doctors prepared to abuse the high ideals of medicine by allowing the healing art to become subordinate to big business. But merely living the other side of the Atlantic, or practising in a country where socialized medicine is limited, does not suddenly turn good doctors into bad ones or men with ideals into unscrupulous predators.

To an English woman, used to subsidized drugs and free medical care (or more properly medical care which *seems* free

F

because payment is concealed within National Insurance deductions), the cost of keeping healthy in the USA could certainly seem pretty high. But I found many instances of compassionate doctors adopting an almost Robin Hood attitude, with the rich patient being used quietly to subsidize the poor patient.

The problems of availability of HRT, of how it can be obtained and financed, will no doubt be solved in different ways in each country. But behind the different medical systems and solutions, all over the world the same pressures are at work.

There is the pressure of numbers, of the increasing *quantity* of women living on long beyond the menopause. And there is also the pressure of *quality*, of the fact that in the main today these are educated women, women trained often to do interesting and demanding work, and wanting and expecting to be kept fit enough and energetic enough to go on doing this work. There is the pressure of communication, of the fact that these increasing numbers of educated women can read, hear and see features on HRT. They know it exists. They believe it can help them.

For their own sakes, for the sake of their families and for the sake of society itself, much more needs to be done in the field of positive health, to extend for men and women the period of mental and physical vigour. And this has to begin by ensuring a healthy middle-age, for that is the time when most of the chronic diseases of later life begin.

Even on existing knowledge and research results alone, HRT promises to be good preventive medicine, not just against the immediate menopause symptoms, but in the long-term against some of the important chronic diseases – against those of the cardiovascular system; of the nervous system, and probably against some forms of malignancy; against osteoporosis, some types of arthritis and against prolapse and incontinence, the scourge of women in old age.

Instead of repeating the parrot cries of 'unproven', which we have heard for so long, it is up to the medical profession to initiate the studies and research necessary to really resolve the remaining questions and fears, so that a true balance sheet can be drawn up on the value of HRT.

Meanwhile enough is known and enough women are eager and available, for the required studies to go forward with truly significant numbers of patients involved.

Medical tradition is against rapid change, hostile to new innovations, and no doubt on balance we should be grateful for this. Only reasonable caution and painstaking research and testing can ensure that tragedies like the thalidomide one are kept to a minimum.

But women now have been on Hormone Replacement for nearly a quarter of a century. The contraceptive pill with its essential oestrogen content has been widely used for well over a decade. During all that time, despite the increased usage of oestrogen this represents, there has been no parallel increase in breast cancer, and cancer of the uterus has declined. In contrast the incidence of lung cancer has soared, showing cigarettes not oestrogen indicted.

In America, quite apart from the convincing survey of Dr Byrd and Dr Burch at Nashville, the prospective screening of 550 000 women entirely failed to establish any basis for a hormonal link with breast cancer.[1] Commenting on this, Dr E. Cuyler Hammond, vice-president for epidemiology and statistics of the American Cancer Society in New York, stated, 'I was sure this disease was hormonal and that with the right combination of questions we would find a pattern that confirmed this. The hormonal theory of breast cancer etiology has been dealt a major blow.'

In Great Britain too, the 1974 reassuring preliminary report of the Royal College of General Practitioners on the contraceptive pill must improve the whole climate of medical opinion toward wider use of oestrogens. The report covers the first six years of a survey involving 46 000 women, to judge the effects both adverse and beneficial of the Pill. It states, 'The risk of serious illness is very small. Use of the Pill brings other benefits besides contraception . . . and it could well be that the beneficial effects actually exceed the adverse reactions.'[2]

In particular the report made the point that there was no evidence that the Pill is associated with cancer of the breast or cervix and may indeed be responsible, if only slightly, for the prevention of non-cancerous lumps and inflammation of the breast, and possibly against the development of ovarian cysts.

It also stated that no evidence had been found that diabetes was acerbated by the oral contraceptive.

The wide publication of such findings by a traditionally cautious body of medical opinion must help to sweep away lingering fears. Subject only to the proviso that oestrogen administration must *always* be cyclic and regularly interrupted, there seems little reason now for doctors to withhold this treatment.

Unfortunately it does sometimes seem that the medical profession tend to be more than reasonably cautious where new ideas to improve the purely female lot are concerned. It must seem almost unbelievable to doctors today, that in the middle of the last century, women were allowed to go on suffering and dying from puerperal fever for twenty years after Zemmelweiss had effectively demonstrated that the infection could be eliminated by the now obvious precaution of properly cleansing the hands before an internal examination. Doctors could not accept such a simple but new concept, even when by using this basic hygiene, Dr Zemmelweiss reduced the deaths in his own Obstetric ward from $11 \cdot 4\%$ right down to less than half of 1%.

Caution can be carried too far. Obviously it is easier for the doctor with any doubts to do nothing. That way he runs no risk of incurring blame. The menopause can be endured. Why involve himself in anything still slightly controversial? That is how many doctors still think and feel.

One American doctor, Francis P. Rhoades of Detroit, Michigan, believes in some cases other factors are also at work. In an article in the *Journal of the American Geriatric Society* in 1967 he urged,

The physician should not let inherent male resentment of female longevity and biological superiority deter him from his medical responsibility. Those who regard the menopause as God's will should critically re-examine the traditional goals of their profession. Because men do not experience the dramatic and often devastating changes represented by the menopause, they have come to regard it as normal for women to suffer the consequences of cessation of ovarian secretion.

All splendid ammunition for Women's Lib! But I cannot believe that in many cases this sort of resentment is really at work. I can believe that apathy is, and to some extent this is the fault of women themselves. Far from making too much fuss about the menopause, in the past they have made too little.

If every woman now genuinely suffering from a miserable menopause took herself to her doctor, made him aware of her problems and insisted on effective medical help, apathy toward the menopause simply could not continue.

But to enable doctors to give this help, they must be educated and medical schools need to put far more emphasis on the menopause. Like contraception and sexual problems, the menopause has been almost totally neglected in the training of doctors. The menopause, its treatment, and the place of Hormone Replacement Therapy, must be given a place in every syllabus of every medical school, and should be included also in refresher courses for older doctors, not only to bring them up to date with existing knowledge, but to *keep* them up to date as new developments come along.

For the future of HRT is likely to include not only more and improved oestrogens, with very specific effects and targets, but also improved techniques. Already for instance, tablets are available which release their contents only very slowly. At the moment this slow release is limited by the time the tablet can spend in the gut. But it may prove possible to coat the hormone at a molecular level, so that it is released into the blood stream over prolonged periods, perhaps to allow a once-a-month tablet.

In the longer term, there may even be artificial ovaries. Already the chemical reactions the ovaries perform to produce their oestrogens are known, and eventually artificial substitutes may be used to synthesize these hormones actually within the body, when the natural ovaries cease to function.

Alternatively some day the genetic engineers may be able to locate and cancel the vital switch which instructs the ovaries to shut down.

But most of this lies in the future; in the meantime I believe the young women of today, used to their daily hormone contraceptive pill, will find by the time they reach the menopause, it will be accepted medical procedure for them to be switched to a replacement dosage of natural oestrogen. It will be as natural to combat this aspect of the ageing process, as it is now to get the eyes tested and be given a prescription for the right lenses. Replacing oestrogen deficiency at the menopause will be as automatic as it now is to replace thyroid deficiency or give insulin.

And maybe when the words 'Women's Lib' are no more than the remembered echo of some old battle-cry from an ancient victory, the words 'Biological Lib' will continue to have meaning for women, as the basic freedom, not designed to deny or decry the female role, but to control and maintain it.

Appendix 1: Mail witness

Letters from my postbag recounting the experiences of ordinary women and ordinary families, caught up in the miseries of the female menopause, provide more convincing evidence than any words of mine, both of the dimension of need and the degree of help required. They also reassure other women that they are not alone in facing certain problems at this time, and this in itself can provide a form of comfort.

Unhappily, with the bulk of my mail coming from British women, many of these letters also bear graphic witness to the difficulties still experienced in the UK in obtaining treatment and the prejudice and ignorance at GP level. But over three years and five thousand letters, there has been a gradual but sustained trend toward a breakthrough, with more and more women reporting success in obtaining treatment and taking the trouble to write and tell me how well it is working and how wonderful they feel.

So this appendix is not written by me. It is written by many different women, most of whom I have never met, but all of whom I thank. A great many of them would have been quite happy for full names and addresses to be published, but others were shy about this because often they had written freely about intimate problems. So it was decided to standardize presentation and in all cases merely use an initial and a place, and also obviously to publish only the really relevant extracts.

'. . . I am very surprised that the Family Planning Association does not intend to extend their services to older women. It seems to be a logical step to treat the menopausal symptoms that often arise in women who have attended FPA clinics for years and are then taken off the Pill. It would seem a natural follow-on to take vaginal smears for hormone levels, in the same way that the cervical smear is already done by FPA doctors . . . this would ensure that all the resources and equipment (and administrative machinery) is used to its fullest extent in a most economical way.

'And speaking of economy, a happy, healthy Gran is far less strain on the NHS than the tired, nervous middle-aged Mum, jogging along through life with the aid of endless expensive drugs such as Librium etc. The hospital beds and nursing staff can be better utilized than for needless results of falls in the home – I refer to the broken hips etc. in older women, which lead to extensive stays in hospital often extending in the future into permanent geriatric care. I do think someone at top level should be tackling the FPA about hormone replacement becoming part of their service.'
Mrs W., Surrey

'How can we get our doctors to take us seriously? I am an ordinary NHS patient, aged forty-three years with three children. I am far from being a hypochondriac and have rarely visited my doctor, except for the babies, in years. Twelve months ago I went to him to tell him I had never felt so dreadful in my life and felt sure I was suffering from some obscure disease. He just laughed and said I was a healthy colour for a corpse.

'Two months ago I went back again, mentioning that I felt physically weak, very depressed and at least twenty years older (my husband says I look it). This time I was told "It was just my age and nothing could be done". I wasn't given any advice so came home and read an ancient book on the menopause. My husband is younger than me and very fit and all this is not helping our marriage. He puts great reliance on medical advice, and if the doctor says there is nothing wrong with me, my husband believes him. Please where can I get HRT?'
Mrs W., Bordesley Green

'. . . Why is it we can read about these things which sound just what we need, but if we ask our doctors they would probably say they have no time for such trivial

things? They give the impression they have really sick
people to attend, and anyone worrying them about the
menopause is just neurotic.

'My periods stopped at thirty-nine and for eight years I
have felt upside down and sometimes have felt like suicide.
I feel I have nothing to live for and I really touch bottom.
My skin has aged and hairs grow round my mouth and chin.
Believe me, this is not just vanity, although I suppose I do
want to look better, but most of all it is the terrible
depression that really knocks me flat and the awful
headaches.

'I am not a neurotic. I am just a woman who has brought
up three children, two are university students. I live in a
council house, have a job and a decent husband, but I
would just like to know how people like me can get the sort
of help you write about.'

Mrs M.N., Essex

1st letter

'. . . While I am grateful to the Press for bringing such
treatment to my notice, please, what is the use if we are
unable to obtain it?

'It is now nine years since I first read about HRT in an
American magazine and since then I've had five years of the
menopause with all the miserable physical symptoms and
depression. I have written to every magazine and paper
carrying articles on HRT asking where I can get help, but
only get the usual reply – medical etiquette forbids them
giving doctors' names.

'Finally I was lucky enough to find a Canadian doctor
working in this country who examined me and put me on
oestrogen. The change was miraculous. However, after one
year, he left and returned to Canada, and his successor
refused to continue the therapy. He gave me a prescription
for sedatives which I have not even had made up, and patted
me on the head as if I were a senile old dear. So here I am
again – insomnia, back-ache, deep depression, the lot!
Can you please help? Don't refer me back to my own doctor,
as I assure you he will not even discuss it.'

2nd letter

'Thank you so much for details of the clinics. I got an appointment and was given the most thorough examination I have ever had; blood tests, urine, heart, lungs, the lot. Above all, it was wonderful to be spoken to as if I were an intelligent human being, instead of a neurotic menopause freak.

'I am now on natural oestrogen and feeling better already. I simply cannot understand the attitude of so many doctors. My original GP never even used the word menopause, but simply told me to get my family to help me over the depression. He made me feel to admit to the menopause was like admitting to being "queer", that it was something which should not even be discussed.'

Mrs A.B., Lancashire

'I am fifty-seven and ceased menstruating in 1967. I suffer with frequent hot flushes which make me feel terrible, but I also have a very peculiar sensation, a really horrible feeling as though something is moving through my veins – I find it hard to explain, and if I ever mention it to my doctor, he only laughs. He has never even asked me about going through the "change".

'My query really is: Have you come across anyone else with this sort of symptom? It makes it worse not being able to convince my doctor or explain how awful it feels. You mentioned on the programme that there are some special clinics. Could you tell me how to find out about them?'

Mrs H., Birmingham

'I work full time in a large and busy school as well as looking after my home, my husband and a twenty-year-old son. I am only forty-four but the menopause seemed suddenly to hit me with "hot waves" so frequent and severe that I would wake up at night soaking. This, coupled with mild cystitis (which I had never had before) was making my life at school and at home very difficult. Now only after a couple of months on 1.25 mg Premarin, it

is wonderful to be entirely free of flushes and feel normal
and healthy again.'
Mrs W., Birmingham

'Since the onset of the menopause life has been very
grim. I am being woken at night with palpitations and night
sweats and also suffer from a type of migraine. I have seen
my doctor but get no relief from the treatment he has given
me, although I take as many as twelve pain-killing tablets a
day.
'The depression and apathy I feel are affecting both my
marriage and my job, which carries a great deal of
responsibility.'
Mrs M.P., Essex

'While living in Canada four different doctors there
prescribed natural oestrogen and it was excellent for me.
Since returning here in April 1972 and running out of
tablets, I have been absolutely up against a stone wall.
'My GP does not agree with it at all and regardless of my
well-being and the fact that I have been so well on it for so
long, utterly refuses to prescribe. It is the more maddening
because I know from enquiries at the local chemist that the
oestrogen I was on, called Premarin, is obtainable, but only
on prescription.
'I have been made to feel positively humiliated for wanting
to stay well and attractive at my age. Yet in the small town
where we lived in Canada, prior to moving to Montreal, all
my friends of my age were benefiting from replacement
therapy and that was seven or eight years ago now.'
Mrs F.D., Devon

'. . . We fifty-plus women work of necessity, not for pin-
money or out of boredom. Our grown-up children are more
prone to marriage break-ups and come back to Mum for
help. After a hysterectomy eighteen months ago, I have been
in poor shape to help anyone or get through my own life.

I just wish each day away. The doctors considered it a successful operation, but for me it has been a disaster, leaving me subject to fearful hot flushes, night sweats and worst of all, deep depression.

'Now I hear of this treatment which could help me and my whole family, who are naturally affected by my condition. Our doctors tell us it is "natural" and advise us to accept it, but why should we? Nothing else is considered "natural" today, why should this particular condition go untreated? At fifty-three I still have so much work to do and my family needs my help.'

Mrs J.H., Middlesex

'. . . My mention to my GP of natural hormones produced a positive sneer and I was told that she had read the article and it was nonsense and there was no such thing as natural hormone. All very scathing and I left the surgery, only too glad to be clutching my temporary reprieve in the form of synthetic oestrogen.

'I had not been able to mention to this doctor some other problems I was facing, such as severe shrinkage of the vagina plus complete loss of sensation in this area. When I ran out of pills again all these things became worse, and I know I became crabby because my fourteen-year-old daughter asked me why I didn't get some more pills.

'So I went privately to the special clinic and my smear showed my own oestrogen was almost non-existent. Since being put on natural oestrogen the hot flushes have disappeared completely, and I feel perfectly well again and able to cope with life.'

Mrs K.T., Middlesex

'I am forty-eight and have started the menopause and I get so depressed. I've been to my doctor over hot flushes and sweating and sleeplessness at night, but he doesn't take much notice, just says it is natural and gives me tranquillisers to keep me quiet.

'I have a job in an office and three children, the youngest

only nine years old, and a dear good husband, whom I love very much but our sex life is rapidly becoming nil because I feel so awful. Please can you help me?'

Mrs M.V., Worcestershire

'. . . I am a State Registered Nurse and my work is demanding. From Premarin I am finding great benefit. I am on a twenty-eight-day cycle with one week off. There are no side effects and it seems to have given me a great deal of energy, although I only heard of it and started on it later than recommended and well after the menopause.

'Judging from my experience and observations over some years of working in geriatrics, I am strongly of the opinion that if the treatment could be made available on the National Health at the right time, much of the degeneration and suffering of old age could be retarded and alleviated.'

Mrs G., Oxfordshire (State Registered Nurse)

'I had great difficulty in getting this therapy. My doctor refused and even when I found a specialist, he would not sign the note to refer me.

'But then I changed to a new doctor (a woman) who approved of HRT and I went privately to a doctor who specializes in it and has given it for twelve years. I think more than special problems with me it was a question frankly of just dreading growing into old age until I have to. I am seventy-three now, but feel fine and look, so I'm told, very much younger. When I had an operation some time ago, for a while I had to leave off the oestrogen therapy and I soon noticed the difference. It really has altered my whole life.'

Mrs E.M., London

1st letter

'I am writing to you in sheer desperation. I can see no future for myself and recently tried suicide, so that my family, my son and my husband, could be free of their trouble and worry about me. My son has just left home, to share a flat with a friend, and I know this is the thing to do nowadays, but I wonder if it has to do with my behaviour.

'I am fifty and with the onset of the menopause, have felt like an old woman, having to give up my job because I could not cope with it as well as my home. Sex is not only painful, but I have no interest in it whatever. My husband and I read your article in *Good Housekeeping* and he said, "This is just you – this is what you need."

'My doctor says there must be some reason for my breakdown (his term), but there is nothing more than I have set out here. My doctor has been giving me up to fifteen pills a day but apart from making me sleep better, there is no improvement. Recently I have been so miserable I have taken consolation when alone all day in whisky. I have told my doctor of this, and been sent to a psychiatrist who specializes in alcoholism.'

2nd letter
'Within a few days of receiving your letter I got an appointment at the clinic. The gynaecologist examined me and said he would be able to help me. I am now taking the oestrogen tablets and already feel much better. I am to go again in a month's time and then again in three months.'
Mrs K., Nottingham

'Some years ago we rented our house to some Americans and the women were horrified to know that no provision was made to give replacement hormones to middle-aged women. I am a State Registered Nurse and have four children whose ages range from two to fourteen. Over the last two years my menstrual cycle has been disturbed; I suffer from pre-menstrual tension and have put on weight around my hips. When I asked my previous GP for some hormones, he told me he believed in the natural menopause, so I did not go again.

'I would like to consult a gynaecologist on a private basis because I have a husband who is very active sexually, and I do not wish to spoil our lives or those of my children with a wife and mother who is under strain. I consider it is much cheaper to treat this condition at this stage rather than let it develop further.'

Mrs S., Berks

'A gynaecologist has put me on oestrogen treatment. I have been feeling much better, but every time I go to my local GP for the tablets, he warns me that not enough is known about long-term results and whether it can produce cancer, which I am sure is no doubt very laudable, but naturally it disturbs me. Could you put me in touch with someone who has been on this therapy for a long time, to reassure me? My GP has made me very nervous but I feel so well, I just can't give up and go back to the misery of hot flushes and sweats.'

Mrs K., Herts

'. . . A year ago I wrote to you in great distress explaining that when I was forty-five I had my womb and ovaries removed, and since then had been in a most miserable state. I was not given hormones but only barbiturates which did nothing but made me feel giddy. All my doctor would say was that I had to expect it at my age. But you don't like to feel you've had it at fifty. Anyway after your letter I went to the gynaecologist and he put me on Premarin. I felt I must let you know how much better I feel. I can manage my housework again and that awful heavy feeling has gone. I am so grateful and must apologise for not writing before. My husband made me write to you the first time because I was in such a state that my marriage and the whole family were suffering. He wants me to tell you what a difference the treatment has made to all our lives.'

Mrs S., London, E.7

'. . . Like a lot of women I have a doctor who seems to feel that Librium and anti-depressants are the answer to all female ailments at this particular time.

'From having a happy married life and being an ordinary individual, over the last three and a half years I have become an anxious, irritable, moody, introspective *thing*. Because of continual irritation in the vagina, intercourse has become a memory, and when my husband and I went together to see our family doctor we were told, "There's nothing I can do about it". I have a really wonderful husband, but the feelings of utter frustration loom larger than life at times. At fifty-three sex is not the vital thing it was when we were twenty-one, but it was always there, but now the discomfort amounting to real pain and the lack of help from the doctor whom I thought could help, has meant our sense of humour like our relationship has become very strained.

'I find it very hard to believe that the present "me" is the same woman who used to sing over the housework, enjoy the family and friends and not have to wonder how things will be in the morning. Will it be an up or a down day? I wouldn't have believed the "change" could be just just that – transformation is a better word.'

Mrs L., Ilford

'After a hysterectomy at the age of forty-eight, when I looked only thirty-eight, I was afflicted with hot flushes every ten minutes day and night. My husband retired to his own room and my marriage was finished. From then on I aged rapidly. My skin dried up and my hair thinned. I get desperately tired. After the operation I know that I must lack hormones, but my doctor will not give them me.'

Mrs L., Canterbury

'I am a nursing sister and cheered you on in your radio talk, nodding full agreement with all you said. From personal experience I know replacement therapy works. I have been on 1.25 mg. Premarin for six months and feel terrific. Now I advise all my apprehensive post-gynae patients that if they can't get oestrogen replacement they

must change their doctor. I had to bombard my own GP before I got it.'
Mrs G., Tonbridge

'As soon as I began to get hot flashes and to feel off colour, I knew my oestrogen level must be down. As an actress, it is vital to feel and look well and I set out to get a test done to check on oestrogen levels, but I found even here some doctors are reluctant to do this and still appear to feel that replacement therapy is not necessary and women should battle on. One doctor I went to actually laughed at me. But I had studied medicine and my two brothers are doctors, so I wasn't going to be put off. Since I have been on oestrogen therapy I have felt great. I don't intend to be a menopausal woman at forty-five or fifty or ever. Now my children are grown up, in fact I am getting back to filming and am quite busy.'
A.C., New York

'I've been on oestrogen since I was forty-seven, when I started to suffer from menopausal symptoms, particularly bad headaches and depression. My doctor put me on Premarin and within weeks I felt fine and it's gone on that way. I've never had any problems since and I am full of energy which spills over from my house and husband into sailing and bowling. I feel sorry for women who don't have this help and I am glad you are campaigning for wider usage. I have one friend now who has to stay in a dark room because since the menopause she keeps getting such terrible headaches. It is all so unnecessary and these women miss so much. Really with families grown up, this is just the time to really enjoy life.'
Mrs D.M., Los Angeles

'I started on oestrogen in 1950 after a partial hysterectomy. At seventy I am still enjoying life with a full-time job as Historian at the Medical School here, working

F

an eight-hour day and driving fifteen miles to work, as well
as running my home. If I run out of my oestrogen tablets,
as I have done just once or twice, I soon notice the
difference. I find myself short-tempered, emotional and
depressed. My regular check-ups show I am in top physical
shape.'

Mrs D.S., Los Angeles

'I am over eighty now and have been on weekly
injections of oestrogen for over thirty-four years. From
May, 1962, this was augmented by tablets to bring the
oestrogen level up. Until quite recently I was not only
active in the real estate business, and treasurer of a local
bank, but Ladies Golf Champion of the New York
Southampton Golf Club. People comment on how little I
have changed and I have certainly kept well and active.
I do not know what I would have done without this therapy
and I feel it should be available to all women.'

Mrs J.S., New York

Appendix 2: Statements and quotes from doctors

'The climacteric is indeed a physiological process and not a disease. The question is where the borderline with pathology should be drawn. In my opinion this borderline is crossed when the woman suffers. The hormonal therapy of climacteric complaints is indicated when the patient consults her doctor for climacteric symptoms and asks for relief.

'Oestrogen therapy in the climacteric patient is one of the most successful and safe treatment regimens. The limitations of hormonal therapy are largely determined by the patient's willingness to cooperate and by the physician's specialist knowledge and experience. Of course, the administration of oestrogens is only substitutional therapy for the climacteric symptoms. The solution of the many social and psychological problems which the climacteric patient has to face at this time cannot be dealt with by hormones. Rejuvenation is not possible either. Nevertheless, treatment with oestrogens can remove many unnecessary complaints, and restore the patient's somatic efficiency and psychic equilibrium. In this sense, oestrogens are a real help for women in the climacteric stage. It should, however, be pointed out that some of the possible long-term effects of natural oestrogen in post-menopausal women have not yet been sufficiently investigated. Furthermore, a possible preventive effect of oestrogens against atherosclerosis and some other diseases of old age has still not been satisfactorily examined and is far from clear. Such investigations are of great importance for evaluating long-term prophylactic treatment and the results will be awaited with interest.'

Professor C. Lauritzen, Department of Gynaecology, University of Ulm.

'Research in the medical field is traditionally more concerned with pathology than with normality. This certainly holds good for the climacteric and the post-menopausal age. In no phase of life, however, is the line between what is normal – and therefore acceptable for the individual – and what is pathological – and therefore unacceptable – thinner than here.

'Finding a solution for the problems of these ages is a medical responsibility, because it is medical science which has prolonged life and, in doing so, has called the climacteric and old age into existence.'

Dr L. Jaszmann, Department of Obstetrics and Gynaecology, Regional Protestant Hospital, Bennekom

'It is not only the dosage that determines the therapeutic effect, but also the dosage scheme as such. Most manufacturers recommend a cyclic administration, i.e. three weeks of medication followed by one week without medication. This is supposed to reduce the possibility of bleedings. What is overlooked, however, is that the latent period between discontinuation of treatment and occurrence of deficiency symptoms is very short, which means that complaints will quickly occur during the days that no medication is given, sometimes even to a higher degree.

'Nowadays, therefore, we advise patients to follow a scheme of six consecutive days of treatment followed by one day without. The advice we give is simple, and easily remembered: Never on Sunday.'

Professor G. A. Hauser, Kantonsspital, Luzern, Switzerland

'I think that our duty is to help our patients to live under optimum conditions. We have, with oestrogens, reached the stage where we know what benefits such a therapy may have. We know a lot about the risks, perhaps not everything. We should not forget that abstaining from oestrogen therapy might harm the patient, and that is also a risk.

'On the basis of our present knowledge of the beneficial effects of oestrogens, it would be wrong to deny these effects to the big group of women in the post-menopause.'

Professor V. Madsen, Gynaecological-Obstetrical Department, Gentofte Hospital, Copenhagen, Denmark

'The decisive role of oestrogen insufficiency in precipitating or accelerating post-menopausal bone loss has been confirmed. In view of the pain, fracture and disability which results from post-menopausal osteoporosis, and its probable relevance to the subsequent high rate of femoral neck fracture in elderly women, a case can be made for post-menopausal replacement therapy with oestrogens on a wider scale than is now generally practised, at least in the United Kingdom.'

Professor B. E. C. Nordin, MRC Mineral Metabolism Unit, The General Infirmary, Leeds, United Kingdom

'Innumerable clinical observations indicate that oestrogens are not only beneficial for the physical symptoms and affect the reactions in autonomic nervous system, but also improve the entire emotional state in the climacteric.

'They relieve general symptoms, such as weakness and fatigue, and purely emotional components, such as anxiety, tension, mood depression and irritability. Furthermore, a great many patients report a general feeling of well-being as a result of oestrogen treatment. The symptoms are rapidly or gradually relieved depending on the individual response and the hormonal dosage used.'

Dr H. Kopera, Department of Pharmacology, University of Graz, Austria

'We have recently started a study into the influence of oestrogens on the quality of memory, the speed of reaction, and the speed of nervous impulses. Our preliminary results show that following castration there are – at least after six months – no measurable changes in the first two. The speed of nervous impulses, however, decreases rapidly after castration. Therapy with estriol-succinate and estradiol-valerate seems to restore the pre-operative level, but the results are only preliminary.'

Professor L. Rauramo, Department of Obstetrics and Gynaecology, The University Central Hospital of Turku, Finland

'Today's society is rapidly changing from a traditional gricultural society into a modern industrialized one. In the traditional society the value of the woman was predominantly determined by her function in reproduction in the widest sense. From this she derived her social value, as a spouse, as the one who gave birth to children, as the one who continued the lineage and the one who reared the children. Her social value determined her personal identity. In this context the end of the fertile period was a major event, perhaps even a disaster. "A partial death", Helene Deutsch says.

'In the modern society a woman's role is no longer exclusively determined by her biological function – this is only one of the aspects from which social value and personal identity are derived. Today a woman has the possibility of a profession and a career, and of social participation in her own right. The end of the fertile period brings changes, certainly, but it means only the necessity of adapting to a new equilibrium.

'Most women know that a treatment for climacteric complaints exists, and many women ask for medical help for their complicated syndrome of complaints. All too often, however, the doctor confronted with the mixture of physical and psychic complaints, recognizes only part of the picture and prescribes tranquillizers. These may, temporarily, curb the symptoms of nervosity which are mainly brought about by the social difficulties, but only procrastinate the adaptation process. It is obvious that this therapeutic approach is only seemingly effective.

'A plea can be made for a preventive therapy with oestrogens for the woman over forty-five, not only with a view to the prevention of climacteric complaints, but also to facilitating her adaption to her new social roles, by bringing – or keeping – the woman in the optimum condition, thus enabling her to cope adequately with the social adjustment.

'The treatable and preventable complaints are the following: (1) the majority of manifestations of the climacteric (2) atrophy of the vaginal wall and related complaints (3) skin atrophy (4) incontinentia urinae in the ageing woman and (5) osteoporosis.

'Such a prevention and treatment of oestrogen deficiency symptoms on a wide scale may be an ambitious plan, but one sometimes has to reach for the stars to land on the moon! The history of medicine has seen many examples of this. Our

ambition should be guided by common sense and a continuous re-appraisal of the value of the therapy.'
Dr P. A. van Keep, International Health Foundation, Geneva, Switzerland.

'We, in our Institute of Social Security in Mexico City, are not in favour of the indiscriminate use of oestrogens. There is no doubt that the patho-physiology of the menopause is an exciting area of investigation, but we must remain objective. We feel that we do not have the final answer to this problem yet. The strong argument in favour of long-term preventive oestrogen therapy to all post-menopausal women is in the claim that it prevents osteoporosis and coronary atherosclerosis. In our opinion this claim has not yet been substantiated by well-controlled studies. On the other hand there is no doubt that some women are in need of oestrogen around the menopause. Such therapy should have a rational basis. It should be highly individualized, and must be directed to the patient and not to the menopause as such.

'It is psychologically important for a woman castrated at an early age to continue to have menstrual bleedings. This is certainly one reason to give both oestrogen and a progestogen.

'When you give oestrogens and progestogens to young castrated patients, the mammary glands remain in better condition than with oestrogen therapy alone.'
Dr Zarate Trevino, Department of Gynaecologic Endocrinology, Hospital de Gineo-Obstetrics No. 1, Mexico

'It is important to decide whether one should aim at prophylaxis or treatment. By the time one treats osteoporosis, for example, a considerable amount of bone has already been lost. It is a case of shutting the stable door after the horse has gone. It is not quite the same as treating the atrophic vagina. Once this has developed one can get a good and quick result with oestrogens. The practice of medicine, as a whole, tends nowadays to be more and more a prophylactic type of medicine. I do not think we should just treat a condition when it arises; we should think more about prevention. That is why I would argue strongly in favour of replacement therapy in connection with the bone disease.'

Dr J. C. Gallagher, MRC Mineral Metabolism Unit, General Infirmary, Leeds, United Kingdom

'Every woman, sooner or later, undergoes inevitable ovarian senescence.

'This phase, the climacteric, is not something she endures for a few months, or a few years, but for the remaining days of her existence – during which time she may well be considered a physiologic castrate.

'The difficulties of the menopause – the imbalance of the autonomic nervous system, the psychogenic disorders and the metabolic disturbances – continue, from mild to severe form, until the end of life. It is unrealistic to withhold measures that may make the transition smoother or prevent disabling pathologic processes.

'Since sex steroids became available, their value in relieving menopausal symptoms is generally acknowledged. There is, however, no unanimity among physicians as to who should be treated or why. At one extreme, the therapeutic nihilist believes the menopause is a physiologic phenomenon which must be managed by reassurance and the use of sedatives or tranquillizers. At the other extreme, others feel that every post-menopausal woman should be given oestrogens, regardless of the presence or absence of symptoms. We think that a more prudent attitude is somewhere between, and that oestrogens are most beneficial in the management of correctly screened patients. No other drug or therapy is able to relieve a menopausal woman of her many discomforts so completely.'

Dr Robert Greenblatt, Professor of Endocrinology, Medical School of Georgia, USA

'Oestrogen is a fundamental hormone in the total physiology of womankind. We have focused our attention too much on the effect of this hormone on the reproductive apparatus without giving adequate attention to its total effect on all body tissues.

'It is estimated that by 1975 more than one-half of the 223 million people in the United States will be women and that women over fifty will make up 13% of the total population.

'The physician has a responsibility to the growing numbers of post-menopausal women in our society. With proper treatment these women can stay youthful, useful, healthy and happy. Properly administered oestrogen replacement therapy will provide a feeling of well-being and eliminate many post-menopausal problems.

'To date there are no known disadvantages to the prolonged use of oestrogens when they are gauged and given in sub-bleeding levels to post-menopausal women. However, it is known that supplemental sub-bleeding dosages of oestrogens prevent degenerative changes in the oestrogens-dependent tissues, particularly the vagina and the perivaginal structure; they also improve the supporting structures throughout the body, particularly the breasts.'

Dr J. Parks, Professor in Chief, OBGYN, George Washington University, Washington, DC, USA

'It is only a question of when and to what extent each woman will become a victim of this insidious (oestrogen) deficiency blended with chronologic ageing.

'Many women may be restored from a chronic state of semi-invalidism to mental and physical health with the judicious use of ovarian steroid therapy. It is unrealistic to withhold measures, before or after the menopause, that can make life pleasant and prevent crippling and disabling pathological processes.'

Dr W. G. Francis, Chief, Dept. of OBGYN, York-Finch General Hospital, Toronto, Ontario, Canada

'Long-term replacement therapy with oestrogen for complete gonadal failure is far more rewarding (than short-term use for symptomatic relief) and should be continued indefinitely to retard the physical atrophic changes and the development of degenerative metabolic disorders. This is an

F*

exciting area of preventive medicine which will help women to retain their good health in their advancing years.'

Dr M. E. Davis, Joseph Bolivar DeLee Professor Emeritus of OBGYN, Univ. of Chicago, Illinois, USA

'Oestrogens generally will relieve all symptoms (of atrophic vaginitis) within a short period and transform the red mucous membrane into a pale, healthy vagina.

'Oestrogen also plays an important role in maintaining the pelvic supports of the uterus and bladder, as well as the mucus membrane of the bladder. The summation of these effects is to preserve all of these structures in a healthy condition, as they are during the reproductive years, and to reduce the frequency of cystitis, stress incontinence, and prolapse.'

Dr E. J. DeCosta, Professor, OBGYN, Northwestern University School of Medicine, Illinois, USA

'Twenty-six per cent of women past the age of sixty have undoubted osteoporosis with vertebral deformity. The minimal dose of conjugated oestrogens for post-menopausal osteoporosis is 1.25 mg. a day prescribed in cycles of twenty to twenty-five days each month.

'When dosage has been established we maintain it; and it should be emphasized that therapy should be continued for the rest of the patient's life. I know of no other way to prevent more deforming fractures. I usually tell my patients that they should continue treatment for at least the next fifty years.

'I should add that patients with senile vaginitis whose dose of oestrogen is increased because of osteoporosis need no longer use vaginal preparations as a method of local treatment. The larger dose of oestrogen required for osteoporosis is more than adequate for vaginitis.'

Dr Gilbert Gordan, Professor of Medicine, UCLA Medical Centre, San Francisco

'Historically, and too often hysterically, oestrogens have been endowed with malignant potentialities. Paradoxically, it has been pointed out that even conservative physicians may not hesitate to give sedatives or tranquillizers, yet they stop at the suggestion of oestrogen replacement therapy. This is baffling to a good many doctors. . . .

'The attitude that "time will tide the patient over" seems to me regrettable, even if symptoms are not too severe. Sometimes moderate or even mild menopausal symptoms, superimposed on the other non-menopausal symptoms, may create a heavier burden than a woman can comfortably bear. . . .

'Even though oestrogens cannot cure emotional problems, a woman is better able to cope with these problems if her oestrogen-related symptoms are relieved or eliminated. . . .

'It is true that many women don't require any therapy and are not truly oestrogen-deficient. However this is of little comfort to those who *are* oestrogen-deficient and *would* benefit from therapy. It's like being reluctant to treat a patient with pneumonia because there are plenty of healthy people around.'

Dr Sherwin A. Kaufman, Consultant Gynaecologist, New York

'For our middle-aged women, accustomed to cyclic administration of natural oestrogens and the added utilization of an appropriate progestagen, there will be no climacteric with its menopause. For these women, in fact, for almost every woman in the civilized world, the climacteric and menopause are unnecessary, totally obsolete. Our older ladies will avoid osteoporosis and their bones will not break. Non-shrivelled breasts and genital organs will be taken for granted. These women will be infinitely more pleasant to live with. . . .'

Dr Robert Wilson, Consultant Gynaecologist, New York

'Many physicians believe that endocrine therapy during menopause affects primarily the autonomic nervous system reactions, not the pyschiatric symptoms. I disagree. Oestrogens improve the entire emotional state of the patient.'

Dr Dorothea Kerr, MD, Payne Whitney Psychiatric Clinic, New York

'With today's longevity most women live a third of their

lives after the menopause. The degenerative processes are therefore a greater problem than they have ever been before. Oestrogens are by no means an elixir or eternal youth, but they can delay many of the most troublesome degenerative processes of ageing in women, and I am certain we are going to see increasing acceptance of their use for retarding the degeneration.'

Dr Patrick Bye, Senior Medical Adviser, Schering Chemicals, UK

'We cannot promise our ladies that oestrogens will restore them to everlasting youth – but we can assure them they will be healthier, happier, more vigorous, and more contented members of our society.'

John W. Walsh, MD, Washington DC, Clinical Professor of Obstetrics and Gynecology, Georgetown University Medical School

'The climacteric syndrome is unique to the human. In no other species in the animal kingdom do we find the complex of symptoms and findings that are seen in the menopausal female. It may well be that the human female, because of the advances of medicine now lives much beyond her reproductive potential consequently she is then exposed to the exigencies of ovarian oestrogen deficiency. It is for this reason that we feel that the climacteric syndrome, whether presenting with or without symptoms, warrants continuous long-term oestrogen therapy; thus one would treat the oestrogenic-deficient female in much the same way one would treat a thyroid deficiency whether or not there is a presenting symptomatology.'

Herbert S. Kupperman, MD, Ph.D., Gynaecologist, New York

'The menopause is a chronic and incapacitating deficiency disease. Its prevention and treatment may well become an entirely new sub-speciality, particularly appropriate for incorporation into general practice. The current availability of oestrogens and progesterones that are potent, effective and relatively safe, provides the physician with the therapeutic agents that will minimize the multiple disorders of the menopause.

'Because of the ever-increasing number of post-menopausal females in our society with the means and desire to preserve their femininity, the medical profession will be under pressure to accept this new responsibility that is being thrust upon them. The widely-quoted fear of cancer as a reason for withholding treatment with hormones is no longer tenable.'
Francis P. Rhoades, MD, Detroit, Michigan

'I have to accept that oestrogen replacement protects against osteoporosis and also against coronary thrombosis and that the incidence of cancer appears to go down. If you ask me whether I would put my wife or daughter on it just automatically, the answer is "No". I believe that all medication is double-edged and so even to prevent certain degenerative processes blanket usage is not justified. We do not know sufficient about the long-term effects.

'If a patient has actual menopausal symptoms, if she is having distressing hot flushes, having to change her nightdress three times a night, or finding hot flushes causing her to blush and be embarrassed at a party, then she should be put on natural oestrogen and kept on it. In fact if she is taken off it the symptoms return and so she is virtually on it for life. There is usually a dosage which can be used without withdrawal bleeding.'
Mr Elliot Philipp, Gynaecologist, London

'All women who suffer from menopausal symptoms should be treated and not just reassured or tranquillized. Provided we can exclude the risk of thrombosis, I would like to see long-term oestrogen replacement therapy, using natural oestrogen, available for them. I feel women should be rising up as a body and asking for this treatment.
Dr Audrey Midwinter, Gynaecologist, Bristol

Twentieth British Congress of Obstetrics, London.
'Hormone Replacement Therapy is increasingly widely accepted in Great Britain to treat symptoms arising from either

natural or surgical menopause, but it is not yet appreciated for its additional long-term purpose of slowing down ageing and degenerative processes. This is an equal justification for its use, but it is not necessary in my opinion, when providing oestrogen replacement for the post-menopausal woman to follow a cyclic pattern or even to deliberately induce bleeding with use of a progesterone.

'The shedding of the endometrium is only of use and purpose during the fertile period, when ovarian function and the ebb and flow of hormones is directed toward ovulation and preparing the uterus lining for the possibility of receiving a fertilized egg. It has absolutely no purpose to serve for the woman who is no longer ovulating. Slow continuous release of hormones through implants gives the body all the advantages of replacement therapy without the inconvenience of cyclic bleeding.'

Mr E. Schleyer-Saunders, Consultant Gynaecologist, London

'I have used natural oestrogen and cyclic combined hormone therapy for patients over quite long periods, for as much as ten years in some cases. There is no doubt it is of immense clinical benefit to some women between the ages of forty-five and fifty-five and does slow down some ageing processes for a time.

'No-one should use oestrogen alone and without interruption day in and day out. Prolonged and continuous over-stimulation of the endometrium can be a factor in producing endometrial cancer. The important rule in oestrogen replacement therapy is that it must be intermittent and I believe the combination with a progestogen is a safer system.'

Sir John Peel, Consultant Gynaecologist, London

'I find that on the whole women resent the menopause and the changes that come with it. The earlier it occurs the more acute these changes are. Prolonged menopausal symptoms (which in addition to the hot flushes may include irritability, depression, insomnia, inability to concentrate, lack of libido, and irrational fears) can place a great strain on a marriage and interfere considerably with work and other routine pursuits.

'The menopause represents a hormonal deficiency, and if you accept this then you accept that it needs treatment like any other deficiency. There is overwhelming evidence of the benefits of such treatment, physically, psychologically and sexually. And there is no evidence at all of any harmful effects. My one reservation is that oestrogen replacement should be cyclic and combined with the use of a progestagen at the end of each cycle. Oestrogens *alone* can cause irregular bleeding and possibly other harmful effects.

'I am sure the attitude of British medicine toward this concept is influenced by the structure of our Health Service and our need to determine priorities.'

Mr Herbert Reiss, Consultant Gynaecologist, London

'In 1952 I took part in the preparation of a report describing the things we found out in a survey on the health of older people living in Sunderland and the surrounding area. I noticed part of the deterioration suffered by older people later in life was due to the decline in the natural hormone output. Later in 1958 trials were carried out over many years at the Maddison Clinic for Preventive Medicine for Older People at Teddington. We observed the benefits obtained from hormone replacement in general health, well-being and the protection it gave against loss of bone with shrinking of the skeleton.

'The results of the research work were published in a number of papers in scientific journals, but it was difficult to persuade the editors of the more accessible medical journals to accept our reports for publication. Hence it was difficult to make the information available to general practitioners, most of whom admit they have little or no experience in the techniques – indeed were against them because of either the lack of instruction in their student days or dissuasion.

'I am happy now to see a growing change in the attitude of practitioners in Great Britain. Many write asking for details of the techniques and a few come to obtain personal experience. Slowly the logic is accepted and there is a growing demand from women themselves which is encouraging doctors to learn more about the methods.'

Dr John Maddison, Twickenham, London

'I believe there is a tremendous future in oestrogen replacement therapy. My concept is simple, and the passage of time will prove whether or not it is correct. Simply stated, I consider the climacteric, the menopausal period and the post-menopausal period to be manifestations of a deficiency disease. I use the term disease specifically to indicate that I do not consider it normal that women should be allowed to continue a life with the absence of a substance which is essential for their normal physiology. My analogy, one would not consider preventing patients with diabetes, mellitis or Addisons's disease receiving the respective hormone replacement therapy, and why should we consider the menopause as anything less than a hormone deficiency disease.

'This particular philosophy is also based upon my belief that during the evolution of man, the onset of the menopause in the female of the species was not subjected to the forces of natural selection which have eliminated so many intrinsic metabolic defects. Obviously by the time the menopause had arisen the woman had fulfilled her part in propagating the species. Indeed, it was quite rare for a woman to reach an age where a natural menopause could occur. I think nowadays that one should differentiate between a pharmacological effect and a physiological effect, when one considers oestrogen replacement therapy, and with the wealth of evidence which suggests that no harm arises from the replacement of oestrogen in physiological dosages, I can see nothing other than benefit arising from the more widespread use of oestrogen replacement therapy.'

Dr Mansel Aylward, Clinical Research Consultant, St Tydfil's Hospital, Merthyr Tydfil, S. Wales

'Loss of bulk and elasticity of the dermis and epidermal atrophy, which may first become obvious after the menopause, are, if they are an isolated phenomenon, likely to be regarded by doctors as the inevitable consequence of ageing. It is easy to think that the desire for treatment is motivated by vanity and leave it to beauty specialists or plastic surgeons. It can indeed be argued that a National Health Service should not be concerned with cosmetic defects. Not only does this view ignore the great distress of mind that the outward signs of ageing cause, it also overlooks the possibility that similar atrophic changes may be occurring in connective tissues elsewhere.

'The simplest indicator of ovarian deficiency is the state of the vaginal epithelium, which can be assessed on the cytology of a lateral vaginal wall scrape. As more and more laboratories become equipped for endocrine cytology the simple approach would seem to be to use this as an objective guide to oestrogen replacement.

'There is no doubt that many post-menopausal women given oestrogens consider that their skin looks and feels younger as a result. The improvement is generally greater and lasts longer than that which follows the local application of oestrogen creams.

'In summary, the treatment of menopausal wrinkles with oestrogens may be justified if the patient is distressed by their effect on her appearance and if there is objective evidence of ovarian deficiency.'

K. V. Sanderson, MB, MRCP, Physician, Skin Diseases, London

'When oestrogen insufficiency develops in a menopausal or post-menopausal female it is permanent, and so far as I know, unless the adrenal begins to secrete increased amounts of oestrogen, this is an irreversible phenomenon. Therefore, when I initiate oestrogenic therapy, I continue it ad infinitum.

'The administration of oestrogen to post-menopausal women with osteoporosis is the most effective and generally accepted treatment.'

Dr R. W. Kistner, Associate Professor of OBGYN, Harvard Medical School, Boston, Mass, USA

'The use of oestrogens during the menopausal years should

be given on the basis of need, as determined by the clinician.
As each patient varies in her own production of small amounts
of oestrogen, one cannot say that each patient requires a
standard dose of oestrogens. The use of the vaginal smear as
an index of oestrogen function for the selection and follow-up
of patients receiving hormonal therapy is, at times, most
useful. This tool, however, is not the only index for intelligent
evaluation of oestrogen replacement therapy. The vaginal
smear is subject to so many extraneous influences, such as
infection, drugs, vitamins, and cardiac glycosides, that its
interpretation, at times, is prejudiced. Patient response to
treatment must also act as a guide in therapeutics with oestrogen.'

*Dr A. F. Goldfarb, Professor of OBGYN, Thomas Jefferson School
of Medicine, Philadelphia*

'At one time oestrogen replacement therapy was dismissed
by British medicine as just something for wealthy American
women.

'Now most responsible doctors and particularly those who
have made any sort of study of it, accept that it is a valuable
treatment, not only to prevent the appalling menopause
symptoms which some women suffer, but also to help keep
them younger.

'I also believe that by delaying the onset of the menopause
it can delay also the onset of cancer and of coronary thrombosis.
But because of the possible complications of bleeding, it must
be given in small controlled doses. With proper supervision
I believe there are no contra-indications, and the cyclic
system of administration is vital.'

Albert Davis, Consultant Gynaecologist, London

'As yet we do not know either the full biochemistry involved in oestrogen replacement therapy nor the full and
possibly long-term side-effects. On balance it is probably a
good thing, but the point is that we do not *know*. Every drug
and every treatment has side-effects and spin-offs which may
not be foreseen. Much more work has to be done properly

to evaluate the treatment, and we have set up a trial for this purpose.

'I am not against the therapy, but I am against its premature widespread use, and against the sort of social and political pressures applied to women and by women, which encourage this. At the present time the GP does not have sufficient evidence either for or against the therapy and cannot yet know how to choose the right oestrogen, the right regimen nor even the right woman.

'The menopause is not only a matter of hormones and changing chemistry. It is a time of changing psychological and social patterns. The woman may need as much help over these as in her hormone status. One-sided management of the whole problem is to be deprecated.'

Professor Philip Rhodes, Dept. of Obstetrics and Gynaecology,
St Thomas's Hospital, London

'My position is that until really controlled prospective trials have been carried out for at least ten or fifteen years, we must treat the concept of oestrogen replacement at the menopause with caution. After all oestrogen has been implicated in deep veinous thrombosis, and also we cannot be really sure about the long-term cancer risks. If and when the benefits are eventually proven to outbalance the risk, then it will be a different matter. Meanwhile it should only be used where the symptoms are sufficiently troublesome to make relief essential. In such cases, apart from temporary help over any short-term crisis, hormone therapy will need to be continued indefinitely or the same symptoms will recur. Long-term therapy is considered to be safer if given as an intermittent course (three weeks tablets with one week clear) with the smallest dose necessary to control symptoms in the individual patient.'

Mr George Pinker, Consultant Gynaecologist, London

'I believe that oestrogens should be used to treat vasomotor dysfunctions of the menopause such as flushes and sweats, but should be discontinued when the symptoms are relieved. Occasionally they may be justified where ovaries have had to be removed in a very young woman or where there is a very early natural menopause. Atrophic vaginitis is of course a specific entity which responds well to oestrogenic suppositories.

'The astonishing suggestion by certain ill-advised individuals that cyclic therapy with sustained menstruation be maintained until the grave is condemned by most gynaecologists. What sixty-year-old woman needs continued menstruation as a "badge" of femininity, especially if she has proved this by having children. Who wants continued menstruation? Can the gynaecologist assume that bleeding in the seventh-decade woman is due to administered hormones rather than organic pathology?

'The use of periodic shedding of the endometrium for life as a means of attempting to avoid cancer of the womb is wishful thinking. Many pathologists believe that in some instances the endometrium that gives rise to cancer contains islands which are not responsive to the progestational hormones, and are not periodically sloughed under the stimulus of this hormone, whether coming from the pre-menopause ovaries or coming afterwards from replacement therapy. Either way, these islands remain constantly under oestrogen stimulation which could culminate in a carcinoma.

'Until there is more conclusive evidence both on this and on the value of oestrogen as a barrier to cardiovascular disease, the use of oestrogens should be restricted to relief of symptoms for short periods. Even the value in osteoporosis is open to doubt, and many doctors believe this is an integral part of ageing. I doubt that oestrogen deficiency is an important causative factor, and in any case to produce any effective brake on bone resorption rates involves such large doses of oestrogen that uterine bleeding almost invariably results. Smaller doses are not effective.

'I deplore the idea currently given far too much publicity that hormones can reduce the inexorable in-roads of age. Endocrine agents are not a panacea for the ageing process, including the menopause, which should be regarded as a physiological phenomenon rather than a disease.'

Dr Edmund E. Novak, Staff Gynaecologist, Johns Hopkins Hospital; Assoc. Prof. of Gynaecology and Female Urology, Johns Hopkins Medical Center

'I am horrified at the thought of looking at the menopause as a disease, and the idea that a vaginal smear with its ratio of mature and immature cells can proclaim a woman abnormal.

'When her reproductive years are over a woman *does* get an "end of the road" feeling. If she is lucky she has the benefit of a good husband, and by that I mean one who understands that it is a difficult time for her and who helps her over her psychological problems. I think the menopause is a time when a woman should be grateful to nature for removing the risk of pregnancy, and if the sexual side of her marriage is well established it should be a time for her to take extra care with her appearance for the sake of her husband and their relationship. I realize of course that many women reach the menopause without the support of either husband or children.

'Oestrogens must not be given indiscriminately to menopausal women to empty the symptomatic dustbin resulting from erring husbands, over-eating, or whatever. If a hormone is used it should be used for specific symptoms.

'I use mild doses of stilbestrol to control flushes and sweating, having completed a very careful gynaecological examination beforehand. Sometimes discomfort at intercourse may require local oestrogen, but I consider that the "maturation index" and similar vaginal cytological tests of a woman's hormone status to be mostly nonsense. Even after removal of ovaries patients do not necessarily require oestrogens.

'Our view here in Birmingham is that symptoms may require treatment but that oestrogens should be used sparingly. The treatment itself may produce unpleasant side-effects such as breast or vulvar discomfort and mucous discharge, and of course any form of steroid replacement may cause post-menopausal bleeding and anxiety. The aim of Replacement Therapy should be to remove the unwanted symptoms without overstimulation of the endometrium. This implies that withdrawal of therapy should *not* cause bleeding, for post-menopausal bleeding spells cancer, or the possibility of cancer, of the womb. This means that all women with such symptoms require full investigation and hospitalization. This is costly, in addition to being vexing for the busy housewife and mother, schoolteacher or secretary.

'To sum up then: the menopause is *not* a disease. It signifies the cessation of menstruation and fertility. Even so "hot flushes" and "sweats", or later coital discomfort, can be a nuisance and the intelligent woman will consult her doctor. In turn he will make a complete physical and gynaecological examination and with circumspection prescribe hormone therapy to cure her symptoms.'

Professor H. C. McLaren, Lawson Tait Professor of Obstetrics and Gynaecology, University of Birmingham

Medical references

The references are presented in the following order: the name or names of the author or authors: the year of publication; the title of the journal: the volume number; further volume reference number (if applicable); page number.

Chapter 4

1. Gordan, C. S. (1973), *American Family Physician* 8, 6, 74.
2. Nordin, B. E. C., Gallagher J. C. (1972), *The Lancet* 1, 503.
   Nordin, B. E. C., Gallagher J. C. (1972), *Clinical Endocrinology* 1, 57.
   Nordin, B. E. C., Gallagher J. C. (1973), *Pulse* 26, 10, 24.
   Nordin, B. E. C. (1971), *British Medical Journal* 1, 571.
3. Aitken, J. M., Hart, D. M., Lindsay, R. (1973), *British Medical Journal* 3, 515.
4. Atkins, D., Zanelli, J. M., Peacock, M., Nordin, B. E. C. (1972), *Journal of Endocrinology* 54, 107.
5. Wilson, R. A., Wilson Thelma A. (1963), *Journal of American Geriatric Society* 11, 347.
   Wilson, R. A. (1964), *Chicago Medical Journal* 67, 193.
6. Villalodid L. S., Buenaluz L., Iledan A. (1973), *Current Medical Research and Opinion* 1, 10, 577.
7. Oliver, M. F., Boyd, G. S. (1959), *The Lancet* 1, 690.
8. Parrish, H. M., Carr, C. A., Hall, D. G., King, T. M. *American Journal of Obstetrics and Gynecology* 99, 2, 155.
9. Rogers, J. (1969) *Pulse* 19, 1, 17.
10. Bailey, C. J., Matty, A. J. (1972), *Hormone and Metabolic Research* 4, 261.
11. McBride, W. G. (1967), *Past-Graduate Medical Journal* 43, 55.
12. Kantor, H. I., Michael, C. M., Shore, H., Ludvigson, H. W. (1968), *American Journal of Obstetrics and Gynecology* 101, 5, 658.

Kantor, H. I., Michael, C. M., Shore, H. (1973), *American Journal of Obstetrics and Gynecology* 116, 1, 115.

Michael, C. M., Kantor, H. I., Shore, H. (1970) *Journal of Gerentology* 25, 4, 337.

Chapter 5

1. Gordan, C. S. (1973), *American Family Physician* 8, 6, 74; (1963–64), *Yearbook of Cancer.*
2. Bakke, J. L. (1963), *Western Journal of Surgery, Obstetrics and Gynecology* 71, 241.
3. Burch, J. C., Byrd, B. F. (1971), *Annals of Surgery* 174, 3, 414.
   Burch, J. C., Byrd, B. F., Vaughan, W. K. (1974), *American Journal of Obstetrics and Gynecology* 118, 6, 778.
4. Nicol, T., Bilbey, D. L. J., Charles, L. M., Cordingley, J. L., Vernon-Roberts, B. (1964), *Journal of Endocrinology* 30, 277.
   Nicol, T., Vernon-Roberts, B., Quantock, D. C. (1965), *Journal of Endocrinology* 33, 365.

Chapter 6

1. Beard, R. J. (1974), *20th British Congress of Obstetrics and Gynaeology, Scientific Programme*, p. 68.
2. Moore, B., Magnani, H., Studd, J. W. (1974), *20th British Congress of Obstetrics and Gynaecology, Scientific Programme*, p. 67.
   Moore, B., Gustafson, R., Studd, J. W. (1974), *Journal of Obstetrics and Gynaecology of the British Commonwealth* 81, 12, 1005.
3. Boston Collaborative Drug Surveillance Programme (1974). *New England Journal of Medicine* 290, 1, 15.
   Report from Boston Collaborative Drug Surveillance Programme (1975), *The Lancet* 1, 1399.
4. Lacassagne, A. (1932), *Comptes Rendus Académie des Sciences* 195, 630.
5. Cutler, S. J., Connelly, R. R. (1969), *Cancer* 23, 767
6. Herbst, A. L., Scully, R. E. (1970), *Cancer* 25, 745.
   Herbst, A. L., Uffelder, H., Poskanzer, D. C. (1971), *New England Journal of Medicine* 284, 16, 878; Editorial (1971), *British Medical Journal* 111, 593.

Herbst, A. L., Robboy, S. I., Scully, R. E., Poskanzer, D. C. (1974), *American Journal of Obstetrics and Gynaecology* 119, 5, 713.
7. Bolton, C. H., Hampton, J. R., Mitchell, J. R. A. (1968), *The Lancet* 1, 1336.
   Elkeles, R. S., Hampton, J. R., Michell, J. R. A. (1968), *The Lancet* 2, 315.
8. Notelovitz, M. (1974), *20th British Congress of Obstetrics and Gynaecology, Scientific Programme* p. 68.

Chapter 9

1. Marmorston, J., Magidson, O., Lewis, J. J., Mehl, J., Moore, F. J., Bernstein, J. (1958), *The New England Journal of Medicine* 258, 12, 583.
2. Rauramo, L., Punnonen, R. (1972), *Frontiers of Hormone Research* 2, 48.
3. Lauritzen, C. (1972), *Frontiers of Hormone Research* 2, 2.
4. Orimo, H., Takuo, F., Masaki, Y., Kazuo, H. (1970), *Journal of the American Geriatrics Society* 18, 1, 11.
5. Jaszmann, L. (1972), *Frontiers of Hormone Research* 2, 22.
6. Aylward, M. (1973), *RCS International Research Communications System* (73–7) 3, 5, 11.
7. Richards, D. M. (1973), *The Lancet* II, 430.
8. Panel on Ovarian Conservation v. Extirpation (1974), *The Menopausal Syndrome* (Ed. R. Greenblatt) p. 186 (Medcom Press, N.Y.)

Chapter 10

1. Wilson, R. A., Wilson Thelma A. (1963), *Journal of American Geriatric Society* 11, 347.
   Wilson, R. A. (1962), *Journal of American Medical Association* 182, 4, 327.
2. Lauritzen, C. (1972), *Frontiers of Hormone Research* 2, 2.

Chapter 11

1. Moore, B., Gustafson, R., Studd, J. W. (1974), *Journal of Obstetrics and Gynaecology of the British Commonwealth* 81, 12, 1005.
2. Lauritzen, C. (1972), *Frontiers of Hormone Research* 2, 2.

Chapter 12

1. Greenblatt, R. B. (1950), *Clinical Endocrinology* 10, 1547.
   Greenblatt, R. B. (1965), *New England Journal of Medicine* 272, 305.
   Greenblatt, R. B. (1972), *Clinician-Med. Gynecology* p. 30.
   Greenblatt, R. B. (1972), *Medical Counterpoint* 4, 15.
   Greenblatt, R. B. (1974), *The Menopausal Syndrome* p. 95–102 and 222–30.
2. Schleyer-Saunders, E. (1971), *Journal of American Geriatric Society* 19, 114.
   Schleyer-Saunders, E. (1973), *South African Journal of Obstetrics and Gynaecology* 11, 32.
3. Hunter, D. J. S., Julier, D., Bonnar, J. (1974), *20th British Congress of Obstetrics and Gynaecology, Scientific Programme*, p. 67.
   Hunter, D. J. S., Akande, E. O., Carr, P., Stallworthy, J. (1973), *Journal of Obstetrics and Gynaecology of the British Commonwealth* 80, 827.

Chapter 13

1. Boston Collaborative Drug Surveillance Programme Report (1974), *New England Journal of Medicine* 290, 1, 15.
2. Royal College of General Practitioners (1974), *Oral Contraceptives and Health* (interim report), Pitman Medical.

Selected bibliography

Wilson, Robert A., *Feminine Forever*, W. H. Allen, London, 1966.
Kaufman, Sherwin A., *The Ageless Woman*, Prentice Hall, New York, 1967.
A Clinical Guide to the Menopause and the Postmenopause, Ayerst Laboratories, Information Pub. Inc., New York, 1973.
Richardson, Robert G., *The Menopause – a neglected crisis*, Abbot Laboratories, Kent, 1973.
Greenblatt, R. B. (Ed), *The Menopause Syndrome*, Medcom Press, New York, 1974.
'Ageing and Oestrogens', *Frontiers of Hormone Research*, Vol. 2, S. Karger, Basle, 1973.

NHS menopause and hormone replacement clinics

Aberdeen: Gynaecology Endocrine Clinic, Dept of Obstetrics and Gynaecology, Aberdeen University, Foresthill

Birmingham: The Menopause Clinic, Professorial Unit, Women's Hospital, Showell Green Lane, Sparkhill

Brighton: The Menopause Clinic, Dept of Obstetrics and Gynaecology, Royal Sussex Hospital

Bristol: Menopause Clinic, South Mead Hospital, Westbury-on-Trim

Edinburgh: Gynaecological Out-Patients, Royal Infirmary, Dept of Obstetrics and Gynaecology, 39 Chalmers Street, Edinburgh, EH3 9ER.

Durham: Menopause Clinic, Dept of Gynaecology, Dryburn Hospital

Glasgow: Gynaecological Clinic, Glasgow Royal Infirmary, Rottenrow, Glasgow, G4 ONA.

Leeds: MRC Mineral Metabolism Unit, General Infirmary

London: Menopause Clinic, Dept of Obstetrics and Gynaecology, Middlesex Hospital, Mortimer Street, W1.

The Menopause Clinic, Dept of Obstetrics and Gynaecology, King's College Hospital, Denmark Hill, SE5.

also The Menopause Clinic, Dulwich Hospital, Dulwich, SE21.

The Menopause Clinic, Dept. of Obstetrics and Gynaecology, Chelsea Hospital for Women, Dovehouse Street, SW3.

also Dept. of Gynaecology, St Thomas's Hospital, SE1 7EH.

Merthyr Tydfil: Dept of Obstetrics and Gynaecology, St Tydfil's Hospital

Nottingham: The Menopause Clinic, Dept of Obstetrics and Gynaecology, City Hospital, Hucknell Road

Nuneaton: Dept of Obstetrics and Gynaecology, George Eliot Hospital, College Street

Oxford: Dept of Obstetrics and Gynaecology, John Radcliffe Hospital

Sheffield: University Department, Jessop Hospital

Index

Compiled by Gordon Robinson